LEARNING YOG

The Beginner's Step by Step Guide

Published by Satya Publishing. For reproduction permission or to purchase additional copies of this book, contact the publisher in writing at 2280 South Monroe St, Denver, CO 80210 or the author through his website at GarryAppel.com.

All photographic images, including the cover, are by the author unless otherwise stated.

ISBN-13: 978-0692993286 (Satya Publishing)
ISBN-10: 0692993282

CAUTION: The practice of yoga is a physical activity that may involve risk of injury to participants. Before beginning any yoga practice, including the activities described in this book, you should make certain you are physically able to do so, including consultation with your health professional in appropriate circumstances.

LEARNING

YOGA

THE BEGINNER'S STEP BY STEP GUIDE

By Garry Appel

Satya Publishing
Denver, Colorado

Acknowledgements

What happens in your life is the product of everything – and I mean all of it – that's gone before. If you could alter or remove even a single event, everything that followed it would change too. Recognizing that, I see this book as the product of a collaboration that has been a lifetime in the making and I truly thank everyone who has been involved in my life thus far. Special mention to a few of the thousands of contributors: to my yoga teachers over the years, Brandy, Karen, Beth, Jeremy, Michelle, Cheryl, Saraphina, Anne, B.K.S. and Tirumalai. To Karen for believing in me, listening to my ideas, proofing and offering kind suggestions for improvements and for providing encouragement and support. To Jon and Henry for teaching me what it means to love. To all my yoga teacher colleagues who have given so freely of their time and energy reading and commenting on the manuscript, making it so much better than I could have produced without them. And to Amy and Rosie for their patience in so beautifully modeling for the pictures in Chapter 6 illustrating the poses. Thank you all for your friendship and dedication to the ideals of Yoga. This work could not possibly have come together without all of you.

Contents

Introduction

So you think you might want to learn yoga.

Maybe a friend or family member has taken you to a class or two and you're interested in learning more. Maybe you've watched a yoga video and are curious. Maybe you have friends who practice yoga and you just want to learn what yoga's all about and whether it might be right for you before you get too invested. More than thirty-seven million people practice yoga in the U.S today and most of those have been doing it for less than five years. People are drawn to yoga to improve flexibility, reduce stress, improve fitness and improve mental clarity. People of all ages practice yoga, split about evenly among the 18-29, 30-39, 40-49, 50-59 and 60+ age groups. Incredibly, more than forty million Americans who don't practice yoga now say they're likely to try it in the next year. If you're part of that group, you're in good company!

The hardest part of trying something new is overcoming the fear of the unknown. My aim in this book is to introduce you to yoga in a very gentle way, allowing it to unfold comfortably a little bit at a time in small easily accessible bits. Instead of starting off with yoga poses, which may seem pretty intimidating, you'll start by getting much more acquainted with your body, experiencing how it works and the miraculous ways it can move and how the parts interact with one another. And you won't just read about these things. You'll experience them, allowing your body to feel and become accustomed to different movements and positions. Each new piece you learn will build on the prior parts and eventually this exploration will come together into the practice of specific yoga poses. This is a big departure from the way yoga is usually taught, as I'll explain in a little more detail below, and that's what makes this book and this approach to learning yoga totally unique. If you follow this path, you'll not only be doing yoga in no time, you'll have a deep understanding of the yoga practice. If you're still with me and interested in digging a little deeper, please join me as we take this wonderful journey together.

I remember my first yoga class very vividly. It was mid-October and Karen (then my girlfriend and now my wife) asked if I wanted to tag along to her Sunday afternoon yoga class at the Monaco Athletic Club. I had never done any yoga, much less been to a formal class, and had no idea what to expect. Yoga seemed vaguely new age-y and I had some impression that it involved contorting your body into pretzel-like shapes. Beyond those vague feelings I didn't really know if it would be physically demanding or more like a gentle walk. So without much thought, it was off to yoga class.

The teacher was an Iranian guy about sixty-five years old named Vali. When we walked in he had already set up his yoga mat at what I assumed would be the front of the room and was taking a small bundle from the pocket of his coat. He carefully began to remove the white cloth that protected whatever was within, like you'd unwrap a precious Christmas present. Inside was a little picture frame, perhaps three inches wide by four inches long. He propped the little picture frame on the floor just in front of his mat. I was curious about what it was and the thought occurred to me that it must be his script for the class. It was only later I learned it was a picture of his revered yoga teacher.

I was attired in my usual workout clothes – knee-length blue Nike shorts and a sleeveless grey top. Karen lent me a mat, which I proudly carried into the room like I knew what I was doing. She set her mat down in what would become the middle row and I put my borrowed mat down next to hers. Eventually, twenty-five people, mostly women and mostly in their twenties and thirties, filtered into the room where the temperature hovered around eighty-five degrees. Some started doing various stretches. Others laid down on their back. Still others sat cross-legged facing the front of the room and closed their eyes, apparently meditating.

Vali spoke with an accent and I found it hard to understand what he was saying. When the class began Vali told us to move into "Tadasana." I had no idea what that meant, but watched as he and everyone else stood up with arms by their side, palms facing forward. I mimicked what he and the other students did. After leading us through some deep breathing for a minute or two, Vali said "Ardha Chandrasana" as he reached his arms up over his head, interlacing his fingers and pointing his index fingers, and began to lean way over to the left in a side stretch.

Again mimicking what he did and looking around to see what everyone else was doing, I followed along as we next bent to the right, holding the pose for what seemed like an inordinately long time. We repeated the bending a few times on each side. I had no idea what "Utkatasana" was as Vali urged us to assume that pose and the slightest bit of panic took hold as he stepped away from his post in front of me and began to move around the room, no longer demonstrating what we're supposed to be doing. At that point the only option I had was to look to what my mat-mates were doing for some clue about how to move. By the time I processed the visual information, Vali and the rest of the class were on to another pose with names like "Garudasana," "Dandayamana Janusirsana" and "Dandayamana Dhanurasana." I perpetually lagged everyone else throughout the whole class by several seconds.

By the end of the seventy-five-minute class I'd worked up quite a sweat, more than I could remember having sweated in any workout before. I didn't know if it was the yoga or the heat or both. Or maybe it was because I was new to yoga and not used to the movements. We'd worked our way from standing and through various balancing poses, to our backs and then our bellies and finally to our seats. We'd bent forward and back and twisted left and right. Although I didn't learn it until later, we'd done twenty-six poses in all, in a practice called Bikram Yoga, and that's all you ever do in a Bikram class – the same twenty-six poses every time. I didn't know then that there were numerous other kinds of yoga classes – gentle yoga, yin yoga, restorative yoga, power yoga, Forrest Yoga, align and flow, to name just a few. I didn't know some classes were heated and others not. I didn't know that some yoga teachers demonstrate every pose and some don't demonstrate poses at all.

I liked Vali's class, even though I was lost most of the time and hadn't kept up. I had been a gymnast throughout high school and a lot of the poses seemed familiar, like what I'd done decades before in competitive gymnastic routines on the rings, the pommel horse and the parallel bars. The next week I accompanied Karen for a return engagement (in part to impress her with my stick-to-it-ness) and then a third and a fourth and a fifth. It wasn't long before I started to attend classes on my own at other places – gyms, athletic clubs, yoga studios and retreats. I experienced many different teachers, different teaching styles and different types of yoga.

My surprise Christmas present from Karen that year was four private yoga lessons with Brandy, one of the yoga teachers whose class I attended frequently and felt a good connection with. Although I was pretty much getting the hang of the yoga poses by then and knew most of the pose names, the one-on-one private sessions with Brandy gave me a much better and detailed understanding of the intended alignment for each pose – where my torso, legs, arms and head were supposed to be – along with the importance of breath. Although I tried to resist, there was something about the yoga that beckoned to me and it wasn't long before yoga classes began to displace my long-standing daily weight training and cardio regime. Ultimately, I was going to a yoga class six days a week. It wasn't long before I began training as a yoga teacher and six months after completing that training I had left behind a career that spanned 35 years and found myself teaching yoga full time.

I learned yoga pretty much like everyone else in the West does – by watching other students and listening to and watching the teacher (if the teacher demonstrated the pose). After teaching countless students, I came to realize that this method of learning – analogous to being thrown in the deep end of the pool and told to figure out how to swim by watching the thrashing of others – wasn't optimal. There are lots of reasons why that's so. For one, imagine you're new to yoga (which you probably are) and you're in a class. You hear the teacher invite you to move into Adho Mukha Svanasana, but the teacher doesn't demonstrate how. First off, unless you're fluent in Sanskrit, you have no idea what the words the teacher just said mean. If you just so happen to speak Sanskrit, you may translate Svan as "dog," Mukha as "face" and you would know that Adho means "downward." Putting that all together, you'd get that the teacher just asked you in a foreign language to move into the pose we call Downward Facing Dog in English. But even knowing what the words mean doesn't give you any idea what you're being asked to do.

Looking at other students might be moderately helpful, giving a general indication that the pose requires you to be on hands and feet with the butt higher than the head, but also leads to confusion. Some students in the class have their knees straight and other are bending their knees. Some have their heels pressing down on the mat and others are up on their toes with their heels lifted off the mat. Some have their elbows slightly bent, while others are straight and still others are hyperextended. Some have their back rounded (curved forward) and others are arched (curved back). Some are holding their head up and lifting their chin away from their chest, while others have tucked their chin towards their breastbone. Even if you happen to have a teacher that models every pose, can you really take in anything but the grossest outlines of the pose by watching the teacher during the class? That would be asking you to look at the teacher, make a mental note of the gross and subtle physical aspects of the pose in a glance, then ask your body to assume the same shape and make adjustments to the shape to conform to what the teacher was doing, all in a matter of a few seconds. A tall order!

Another reason this method of learning isn't optimal is that from their very first contact with yoga and during the earliest and most formative experiences, the student's attention is directed outward and away from their physical and mental selves. Yoga becomes, at least at first, an other-directed activity in which movements are dictated by what's occurring "over there." The student is watching, using their eyes to see what's going on around them and then doing a lot of cognitive work, processing what they're seeing and attempting to synthesize the different ways others are performing the pose into a general rule about where each part of the body should be and then applying those rules to their own body – all in real time. As the student becomes more proficient at yoga, they are instructed to "move inward," internalizing the practice. It's a switch that many people can eventually make. But it's one that's unnecessary, unintentionally leading students off the path in the first instance and then requiring a significant redirection later on, moving from an outer-directed focus to an inner-directed one.

Finally, the "learning by watching" method often results in improper outcomes when people incorrectly think they've got the alignment right, maybe because they're copying their pose after the wrong models or maybe because they aren't aware what shape their body has assumed. An obvious example that most yoga teachers see every day is plank pose. Ideally in plank pose the heels, hips, shoulders and head are all in a straight line, like a flat board. But in any given class you'll see some students in a sort of inverted wedge with their hips lifted above level. Others may have their hips dropped down below level. You'll frequently see students lifting their head up and looking forward in plank, while others have their head dropped down. For many this isn't just a problem of not knowing where their body parts are in relation to one another – it's instead a fundamental misunderstanding of what the body alignment is supposed to be in the pose.

Realizing the potential shortcomings of the way I and most everyone else learned yoga, I spent a lot of time thinking about and working with new students to explore how we could do a better job of teaching. I looked at many books targeted at teaching yoga to beginners and noticed they were fundamentally all the same and took the same approach to teaching yoga as I've described above. Each describes particular poses and teaches the reader how to do the pose. One book takes the student through 60 "essential" poses. Another describes 50 poses that must be mastered to do yoga. Others work from 40, 30, 25 or 10. It eventually became clear to me that the teaching approach followed in the beginner yoga books, as well as at in-person yoga classes and in online videos, is completely backward. The yoga poses and the practice that incorporates the poses are the end result of the learning process. They aren't and shouldn't be treated as the starting point.

The result, which you'll find in this book, is a new approach to learning and understanding yoga poses – a new way of looking at and thinking about the poses. So instead of beginning with yoga poses, we'll begin by examining the component parts of the body and how each of those parts can move and be positioned – what they are and aren't capable of. With that knowledge we'll explore the main shapes the human body can assume, which are basically just three – straight, hinged at the hips and curved. We'll then examine how those basic three shapes can be positioned in space and discover that the options are limited to upright, upside down, face up, face down and on the side. Finally, we'll deepen our understanding by looking at the differences in position that will result from the way we position arms, legs, torso and head.

You're going to do more than just read about this stuff. Yoga is about learning through doing and you're going to deeply integrate the movements and understanding of your body into your very being by working through Practices along the way. Each Practice will focus on something simple and straightforward, like standing upright to notice what that really feels like. Once you've worked through all the Practices, we'll bring it all together into particular yoga poses and you'll learn the poses in a way that lets you understand exactly what each one looks like, based on basic body shape, body orientation in space and leg, arm, torso and neck positions. Only at that point will you learn the name of each of these poses. When you're done with the program, you'll not only have a good repertoire of yoga poses, you'll also have a deep understanding of your body and be able to easily learn new poses as you continue your yoga practice.

This book is my humble effort to share this improved teaching method with the community of prospective yoga students, as well as with current students and yoga teachers. If you're new to yoga and looking for a simple and straightforward way to learn, I think you'll find the approach in this book very accessible and a great way to begin the practice on the right foot (pun intended). If you've practiced yoga for a while, I think you'll find the approach described in this book as a wonderful supplement to what you've already learned and a helpful guide to continuing your practice with confidence and stability. And if you're a yoga teacher, the book will give you a detailed explanation and understanding of my teaching method and give you all the tools you need to share it with your own students.

There are lots of pictures in this book to illustrate the words. You'll meet different models along the way. Block of Clay will be your first visual teacher who will help illustrate the human body and how it works. As we explore more deeply, you'll meet Mr. Yoga who will demonstrate more complex and subtle movements and positions. Finally, when we come to learning specific poses, which you'll encounter in Chapter 6, two human models will provide the visual guidance needed to understand the poses. I am deeply grateful to all four models who have quite literally allowed me to see in ways I otherwise would not. Like all of us, each model has different strengths and challenges and, like my students, I would never ask that they force themselves into a position beyond their unique physical capabilities and limitations. Each is an individual and their modeling of the shapes and poses is unique to them.

I had that exact idea in mind last week when a woman who was new to one of my classes and new to yoga came up to me after class and apologized for "not being able to do yoga right." She explained: "I'm just too fat to move like that." I replied that "there's nothing to apologize for." Remembering a similar conversation I'd had with a different student a couple of years before, I continued: "Did you notice the woman on the mat next to you in class?" "You mean the elderly woman," she replied, "she was really great at yoga." "Yes," I said. "Mary's 71 now. When she took her first yoga class two years ago she couldn't even get down to the mat on her own to sit. She literally huffed and puffed with every simple movement. She's been to class twice a week since that first day. She's strong and supple. The yoga has changed her." Just then Mary happened by on her way out the door and said to me: "thanks for class." "You're welcome. How was your practice today," I asked. "I practiced just how I was supposed to today," she replied. As Mary walked out the door I said to the new student, "Come to class next Sunday and we'll practice again."

This book is a practice guide that you can follow to learn the basics of the yoga postural practice. The yoga poses are called "asana" in Sanskrit, one of the ancient languages of India. In each separate portion of the book I discuss a particular concept and then provide a group of actions – practices – for you to perform so your body can experience whatever has been discussed. The practices are really the essence of my teaching method. The reading preceding the practices is just the setup. My suggestion is that you read through each individual practice and then perform it once, twice, three times or more, before you move on to the next one. Practice until you feel like you've gotten the point of the practice. Also, to get the benefits of this teaching system, you need to take the time to physically work through each practice instead of just reading it through and thinking you get the point. Learning the yoga poses isn't an intellectual exercise. It's a physical practice that eventually allows you to come to know your body – and eventually your mind – in ways you've probably never imagined. The physical practice will allow your body to "feel" the poses and the movements. That's crucial to learning yoga. So don't short-change yourself by rushing through or taking shortcuts. Take the time to really do the practices and I promise it will pay big dividends down the road, allowing you to gain a much deeper understanding of Yoga. Of course, doing the poses doesn't have to be the end of the journey. Instead, it can be just the beginning of a wider exploration of the system and science of Yoga that includes introspection, observation, contemplation, meditation and – ultimately – clear understanding of the world. Think of the poses as the entry point for your practice of Yoga. Once you learn the poses you can, if you want, explore what more Yoga has to offer you.

I am so happy you have found your way to my work and hope you find it helpful and illuminating. I end this introduction the same way I end every yoga class I teach, with the Metta chant:

> *May you be happy*
> *May you be well*
> *May you be safe*
> *May you be peaceful and at ease.*

Namaste.

Garry Appel
September 2017

Chapter 1 – The History of Yoga

To understand the context in which yoga poses have arisen, let's take a very brief look at the history of yoga. You'll often hear that yoga is an ancient practice dating back 5,000 years or more. That story is presumably intended to leave you with the impression that the yoga we practice today has a deep and very old pedigree and that it's worth investigating because it has been around for so long and proved its value. In truth, we know surprisingly little about the history of yoga. However, we know enough to say definitively that the yoga we practice today in the western world would be unrecognizable to a yogi from the distant past. When we hear "yoga" today we think of a type of physical activity involving bodily movement, often flowing movement, from one pose to the other that takes place over a set time, often an hour.

While some ancient texts on yoga survive, there aren't really that many. The Yoga Sutra is the best known of them. It is attributed to an Indian named Patanjali. We don't know anything about Patanjali himself and even the date the Yoga Sutra was written is lost in mists of time. Some scholars date it as early as 500 BCE, while others say it didn't come into existence until as late as 300 CE. Regardless of who wrote it or when, the Yoga Sutra is the most widely read and studied book on yoga that there is. The Yoga Sutra was written in Sanskrit, an ancient language of India. In it, Patanjali describes Yoga as a system that the practitioner can follow to achieve enlightenment. This road or path consists of eight parts (usually translated from Sanskrit as "limbs"). The limbs include moral and spiritual guidelines, breathing practices and various stages of meditation, ultimately leading to Samadhi or enlightenment. It isn't at all clear that ancient yoga involved much movement at all.

The Yoga Sutra identifies the third limb of the Yoga system as "asana," which is usually translated from Sanskrit as meaning to "sit down." It was an important facet of the yogic system because it was through sitting in a still and comfortable posture that the devotee would move into meditation and it was through meditation that union with the divine, Samadhi, could be found. It may be a surprise to you that Patanjali didn't describe any specific postures or asana in the

Yoga Sutra and we know very little about the asana that existed in the most ancient times. The earliest postures were probably few in number and almost certainly consisted of little more than different ways of sitting in meditation. It also seems likely that the ancient yogis didn't practice any sort of postural movement of the kind we think of today as "yoga." It wasn't until many years after the Yoga Sutra that yoga texts started to mention specific poses. Some texts identify as few as seventeen asana and others claim there were as many as 8,400,000 poses.

What we do know is the postural practice has become ascendant, even to the point that for many people the word yoga signifies physical flowing movement and they know little if anything about the other seven limbs of Yoga. We can be sure that the number of asana regularly utilized in the postural practice has certainly increased over the last century. Today, common listings of yoga poses suggest about one hundred basic poses in regular usage, along with numerous variations on those basic poses.

We probably owe the ascendancy of the postural practice to some vagaries of Indian history. At the beginning of the 20th Century, the broad spiritual practice of Yoga had nearly disappeared in India. In the mid-1500's Jesuit Portuguese monks traveled to India as missionaries and strongly condemned Yoga. The Portuguese Inquisition in India followed the monks and sought to convert the largely Hindu population to Christianity. During that period, which lasted into the mid-1700s, the practice of Yoga was banned and, if discovered, often resulted in the practitioner being burned at the stake. British colonial rule, the 200-year period from about 1750 to 1950, followed. In that time, Yoga was seen as part of pagan Indian culture which the British endeavored to replace with their own values. It is thus a small wonder that Yoga in any form survived through this long period.

The yoga we have today can be largely attributed to a revival that began in the early 1900s and can be traced mostly to one man. Born in 1888, Tirumalai Krishnamacharya revived the lost Yoga practice and took it in new directions. Influenced by a movement during his youth to revive Hindu culture and traditions, Krishnamacharya studied the ancient practice of Yoga from an early age. As he told the story, he went on a pilgrimage at sixteen to an ancestor's shrine and had an extraordinary vision: "He found an old man at the temple's gate who pointed him toward a nearby mango grove. Krishnamacharya walked to the grove, where he collapsed, exhausted. When he got up, he noticed three yogis had gathered. His ancestor Nathamuni sat in the middle. Krishnamacharya prostrated himself and asked for instruction. For hours, Nathamuni sang verses to him from the Yogarahasya (The Essence of Yoga), a text lost more than one thousand years before. Krishnamacharya memorized and later transcribed these verses." The roots of Krishnamacharya's teachings are found in those verses.

Beginning in the early 1930s, Krishnamacharya developed what came to be called Ashtanga Vinyasa Yoga, which incorporated gymnastics brought to India by the British colonizers with the perhaps two dozen Yoga poses Krishnamacharya had learned as a young boy. The result was a flowing and dynamic practice that was coordinated with specific breathing (called pranayama in Sanskrit). Several well-known students of Krishnamacharya traveled to the west and spread this new type of Yoga, including one of the very first women Yoga students and teachers, Indra Devi, who in 1955 authored the best-selling book on Yoga, Forever Young, Forever Healthy. For the most part we have these twentieth-century teachers to thank for what we now recognize as "Yoga."

The Yoga of today is neither better nor worse, neither more nor less, than the Yoga of several millennia ago. Yoga has changed and evolved and adapted over the ages. I've included this brief history so you don't have an idealized view of Yoga and instead understand that what we practice today, while it has ancient roots, is very much a product of the modern age. Understanding that context, let's next take a fresh look at the instrument you're going to use to perform the poses, the human body, and learn to think about how the body moves. That will give you a much better and grounded understanding of what the poses are and how your body will be arranged in each pose.

Chapter 2 – Understanding Body Mechanics

Can you visualize this block of clay as something like the broad general shape of the human body? It's about four times taller than it is wide and quite a bit wider side to side than it is deep from front to back. Of course, if we're going to endow the Block of Clay with a more human form, we'll need to add some refinements.

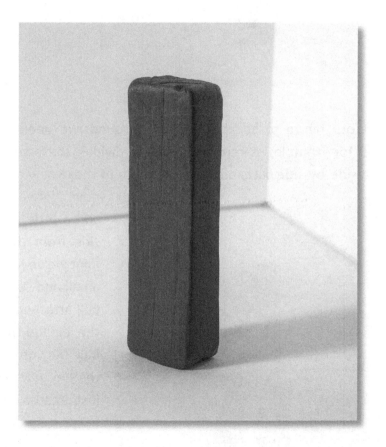

First, imagine that we introduce a way for this form to bend forward, roughly at a point half-way between the top of the figure and the bottom. It would look the picture on the next page.

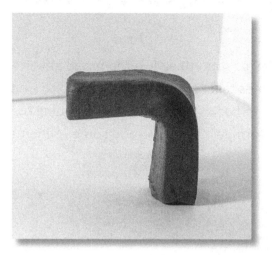

We've of course just invented hips. Notice how the upper half of the figure is still straight. And notice the same is true of the lower half. Literally, all we've done so far is give our model, Block of Clay, a way to bend forward in the middle.

If we want our figure to be able to move around, we need a method of locomotion. Just for example, let's create a biped by dividing the lower half of Block of Clay into two side-by-side parts and allowing each of these new appendages to

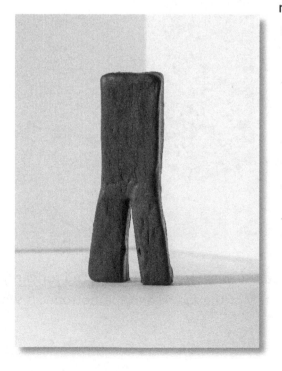

move forward and back and a little bit out to the side from the hips. The joint we've just invented is a ball and socket, with the ball attached to the top of the leg and the socket the ball fits into attached to the hip. We've of course just created legs – straight ones.

Now let's let each of the legs bend roughly in the middle and we can name those bends "knees." This bend will just allow the bottom of each leg to hinge backward. The knee doesn't hinge forward at all. The most movement it's capable of is to allow the leg to return to the straight position.

Block of Clay can now perform locomotion, more or less, by trundling around pretty awkwardly. Many tasks our figure will want to perform in life will be aided by appendages at the top of the body that aren't always occupied with having to stand or walk around. Let's

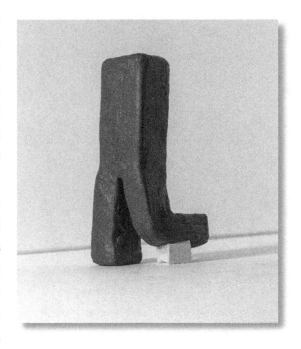

create those from the space above the hips and elongate them a bit so they can hang down past the hips.

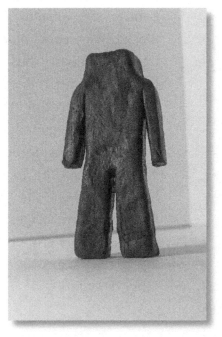

Voila! We've just created arms. Now it would be nice if these arms could move all around – forward, back, up and out to the side. So, we can use the same sort of ball and socket joint we used for the legs. With that joint, our figure can make lots of motions with its arms, including reaching down, shown to the left, and the various motions shown in the two pictures on the next page.

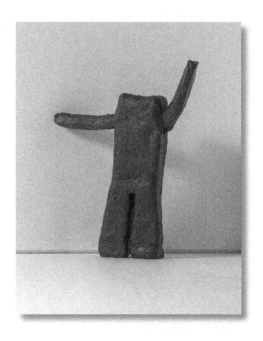

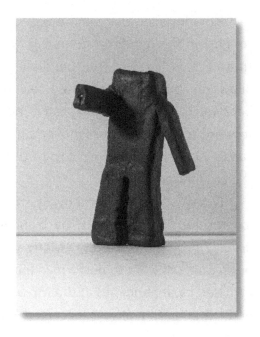

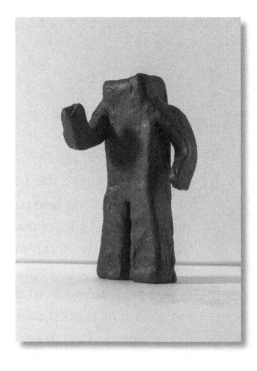

Like the legs, it would be pretty useful if the arms could bend in the middle. That way Block of Clay could pluck berries from a blueberry bush without having to move the whole body and perform a lot of other useful tasks. So, let's give each arm the same kind of hinging joint that we gave each leg. The joint is about half-way down the arm and notice the arm hinges only one direction – forward, pretty much like the leg, except it hinges the other direction.

Now we need something to house a brain to direct all these new motions and some sensory receptors to perceive what's going on. For that let's create a head at the top of Block of Clay and allow the head to swivel side to side and forward and back – pretty much a full range of motion – on a wide tube we can call a neck.

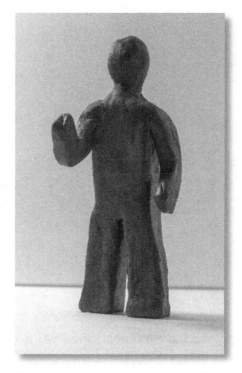

We've left out some subtleties and refinements – hands and feet and toes and fingers – and we haven't completely described all the motions the torso and appendages can move through. But from a broad perspective, what we've done is create a generalized representation of the human body. Now let's see take it for a test drive and see what it can do.

As we saw at the beginning of this Chapter, Block of Clay can hinge forward at the hips and bend to about 90-degrees. In that bend, both the lower and upper parts of the figure stay pretty straight without much rounding or arching. It's fairly easy for Block of Clay to hinge at the hips in a range of motion from straight up and down to 90 degrees.

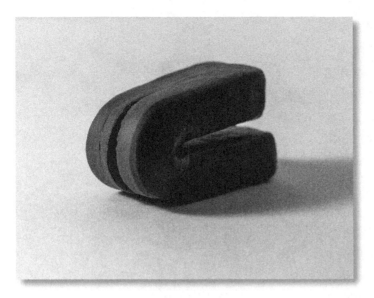

We might continue to fold Block of Clay forward in the middle until it folds completely in half, like in the picture at left.

In practice, because of the way the legs are attached to the torso at the hips, it isn't very easy to fold over completely and keep the back completely flat. So you see some rounding in this configuration.

A subtlety we haven't mentioned yet is that the upper part of the figure isn't static, but can bend forward – rounding – and back – arching. One of the consequences of that ability is that the figure can bend its torso forward by rounding instead of or in addition to hinging at the hips.

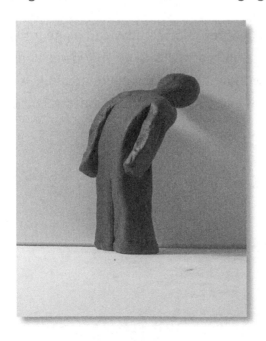

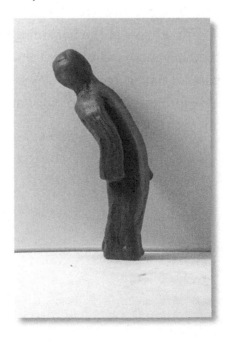

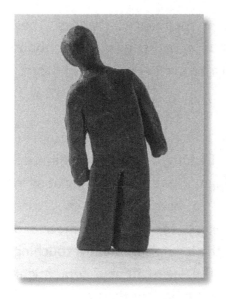

In addition to rounding the back and arching, shown in the last two pictures on the prior page, Block of Clay can curve the upper part of his figure to the side, as shown in the following picture.

Let's pause for a minute and review what we've seen so far. Our figure can be straight, that is not bent at the hips. It can also hinge forward at the hips. Finally, it can round the torso forward or back and from side to side.

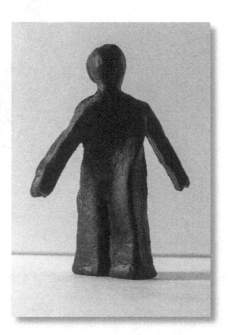

Now let's add a new feature – twists. Block of Clay's torso can twist right or left, moving to something like ninety degrees.

Besides the torso, the head can twist side to side too.

Now let's take a more detailed look at the lower appendages, the legs. They can pivot forward at the hips through a range of motion that ends up being about 150 degrees, as well as out to the side and back. The legs can also twist to a degree.

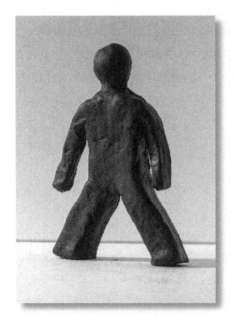

There's one more movement to examine with the legs – bending the knees. The knee joint is just a hinge. There's no twisting at all in the knee joint. So, with the body otherwise straight, our figure can bend a knee and eventually fold the leg up completely, touching the bottom of the leg (where a foot might eventually go) to the back of the upper part of the leg.

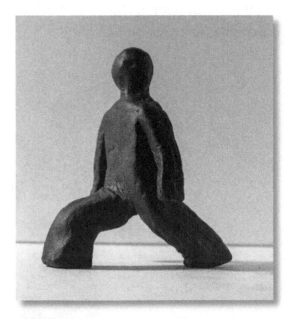

The knee can move through this 180-degree range of motion, more or less, but note that the knee does not bend the other direction. Of course, the legs can move independently of one another, producing lots of different possible combinations. The legs can move in tandem. One leg can pivot out to the side while the other stays straight or both can pivot out. If both legs are pivoted out, the knees on one or both legs can be bent. These are just a few examples of the nearly limitless combinations.

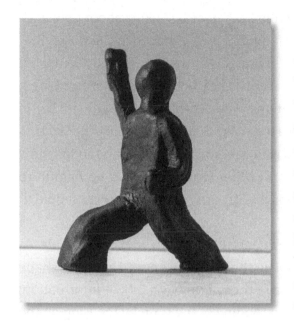

Finally, let's look at the arms. They actually have a greater range of motion than the legs. They can reach up from the shoulder joint, either bent or straight and symmetrical or not. They can reach out to the side, again, with elbows bent or straight and symmetrical or not. They can reach down with elbows bent or straight or back. The picture at left is an example. The right arm is straight and reaching up, while the left arm is reaching down with the elbow bent at 90 degrees.

Block of Clay started life as a simple undifferentiated block. From that, we've created a figure who's constructed the same on both sides (bilaterally symmetrical). 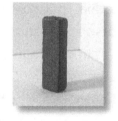 There are just four main joints on each side, a shoulder, a hip, an elbow

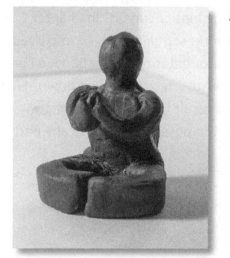

and a knee, and our figure is capable of bending and twisting along the torso above the waist and at the neck. From these basic articulations, endless combinations are possible that will each produce a unique combination of positions, ranging from the straight form we began this Chapter with to a crazy pretzel-like fantasy, such as that shown at left.

On a physical level, each yoga posture is made up just that way – a specific configuration or placement of the different parts of the body oriented in space in a particular way. Mechanically, we can describe each pose by talking about how each part of the yogi's body, the torso, legs, arms and head are placed in the pose. But, from what we already have learned, it's pretty clear that the human body is capable of nearly infinite variations and trying to describe a particular pose by describing it based on a constellation of infinite variations would be pretty daunting. So, in learning yoga it would be helpful to have a way of grouping poses together so that knowing which group a pose is part of will give us a shortcut to understanding how the body is to be positioned in the pose. In other words, it would be helpful to know which poses are like other poses and why. It turns out that's pretty simple to do.

To understand a yoga pose all we really need to start with are two basic pieces of information: what is the basic body shape in the pose and how is that body shape oriented in space in the pose. Once we have those two basic bits of information, we can complete our description and understanding of the pose by focusing on the details that come from differences in how the arms, legs, feet, hands, head and torso are positioned or bent or twisted. It's really that simple.

In the following three Chapters, we'll examine each of those variables. In Chapter 3, we'll examine the basic body shapes found in yoga poses and we'll see that there are just three – straight, hinged at the hips or curved. In Chapter 4, we'll explore the different ways the body shapes whether straight, hinged or curved, can be oriented in space. As with body shape, the orientation of the body in space is easily categorized as upright, upside down, sideways, face up or face down. Finally, in Chapter 5 we'll dive into the variations that result from the way the arms, legs, feet, hands, head and torso are positioned in the pose and whether any parts are bent or twisted.

Practices

In this Chapter we've explored how a generalized human form is shaped and put together and how each of its component parts move at the joints. In the following series of Practices we'll apply that information.

Practice 2.1 – Body Scan. Note: I have created a video of this Practice which you are welcome to use. You can find it on YouTube by searching for "GarryAppel Yoga" and then select the video titled: "Learning Yoga – Practice 2.1 – Body Scan." You can also find a link to the video on my website at GarryAppel.com under the Yoga section. Alternatively, you can record the narrative below on your own and play it back while performing the Practice or have someone read it to you.

Begin by lying down on your yoga mat. If you don't have a mat yet, lie down on a carpeted floor or rug, something that's not too hard and has a uniform surface that won't distract you from the work we want to do. Lie on your back, face up, with your legs straight and your feet about hip-width apart. Your toes can flop out to the sides a bit if you want. Your arms should be straight and by your sides and your palms can be either face-up or face down. Let the back of your head rest gently on the mat. Make sure you aren't lifting your chin away from your breastbone (the sternum) or tucking your chin towards your sternum. Gaze up at the ceiling directly above your face. Now close your eyes softly and inhale slowly through your nose to a count of four or five. Feel your abdomen expand slightly as you breathe in, but don't force the in-breath. Once you feel full, slowly breathe out. Repeat the inhale-exhale cycle a few times until you feel your body settling softly and letting go.

With eyes still closed, begin to visualize your body as a whole. Imagine it resting on the mat, long and straight. Imagine the breath flowing into your body and then out. Imagine your heart beating in your chest and see if you can feel your heart beating every second or so. Can you imagine your heart pumping blood through your arteries to every part of your body and the blood flowing back to your heart through your veins? Now let your attention rest on the big toe of your right foot. Visualize the toe and imagine the bones that make up the toe, without getting caught up in how many specific bones that might be. Let your attention move to the second toe, maybe wondering whether it's longer or shorter than the big toe, and then to the third and fourth toes and then to the little pinky toe. Let your awareness travel up the right foot, imagining the top of the foot and the bottom. Bring your awareness to the heel of the right foot and then to the ankle. Shift the attention to the left foot, beginning with the big toe and working your way up to the ankle, just as you did on the right foot.

Let your awareness rise from the ankles of both legs to the calf on the back of the legs and spiral around to the shins on the front of the legs. Eventually your attention comes to the knees. Pause for a moment and visualize the knees as the point where the two lower leg bones, the tibia and fibula, come together and meet the upper leg bone, the femur. There's a round disc of bone on the front of the knee joint called the patella or kneecap. Imagine it held in place by muscle fibers protecting the knee joint. With your attention rising from the knee on both legs, begin to visualize the long thigh bones which have a ball-like structure at the top end. Imagine that ball fitting into a round open socket on the pelvis to form the hip joint, one on each side of your body. The spine or backbone attaches to the top of the pelvis. It's composed of twenty-four unfused individual vertebrae that get progressively smaller as you move up the spine. Visualize each individual vertebra, one stacked on top of the other. The lowest vertebrae make up the lumbar part of the spine – the low back. Feel the lumbar vertebrae curving gently away from the floor you're lying on and towards your navel. The next part of the spine is the longest. It's called the thoracic. Follow it up and feel how it curves towards the floor. Continue allowing your attention to rise up the spine, coming to the cervical portion that's within your neck and feel how it curves gently away from the floor and toward your throat.

Now become aware of your rib cage, visualizing how the ribs attach to the vertebrae and then arch forward, encircling the upper part of your torso, meeting at the breastbone. Imagine the heart and the lungs, breathing and pumping blood, all encased and protected by the rib cage. Imagine the upper bone of each arm, called the humerus, attached at the shoulders to the top of the torso. Visualize how these joints are similar to the joint between the pelvis and the legs. Let your awareness travel down each arm to the elbow, where the lower arm bones, the ulna and radius, join the humerus and notice how similar the elbow joint and knee joint are to one another. As your attention comes to the wrist, visualize how the bones of the fingers attach to the lower arm bones at the wrist. Finally, bring your awareness back to the top of the spine and imagine your skull attached to the spine and visualize the brain protected by the skull and attached to the rest of your body with a network of nerve fibers that run down the middle of the spinal column, eventually branching out to the arms and legs and fingers and toes.

Once you've completed the scan of your body, breathe in slowly through your nose and imagine the breath flowing away from the toes, up your legs and torso and then out your mouth. As you exhale, visualize sending the breath all the way down to the tips of your toes. Repeat the inhale/exhale cycle twice more and then allow your eyes to open gently and slowly come to a seat.

Practice 2.2 – The Hip Joint. Part 1 - Stand with your back against a wall, making sure the heels and the glutes on both sides of your body are lightly touching the wall. Pick your right foot up, bending your right knee as much as you can. Making sure the glutes, especially the right one, stay grounded into the wall, bring your hand to the right knee and press the knee to the left as much as possible without causing strain. Then bring the knee over to the right as much as possible. Now begin to move the knee in a big circle, up (hugging it into your chest if you can), then left, then down, then off to the right. Ignore the lower part of your leg and begin to visualize the ball and socket joint that connects your leg to your pelvis. Imagine the ball at the top of the leg as it rotates in the socket in the pelvis and become aware how the upper leg bone, the femur, can move relative to the pelvis. Move the femur in circles a few times one direction and then go back the other direction a few times. Notice that you can press your knee off to your right quite a bit more than you can press it to the left (assuming you keep pressing your right glute into the wall) and notice you can press your knee down more (if you let your knee straighten) than you can lift it up. Release your right foot to the floor and then repeat the Practice on the other side in the same way.

Part 2 – Lie down on your back on your mat with both legs straight and the feet about hip-width apart. Ground the right glute into the floor, making sure you don't lift it up off the mat. If you have a yoga strap, you can use it for this Practice. If not, use a heavy rope about six feet long or a long scarf or towel. Holding one end of the strap in each hand, bend your right knee and put the middle of the strap on the instep of your right foot and then straighten your right leg so the sole of the foot stretches up to the sky. Transfer both sides of the strap to your right hand and bring your left hand to the floor beside you, reaching your left hand out to a T. With your right knee still straight, allow your right leg to move off to your right, using your left hand for balance. Depending on your flexibility, you may find your right foot will reach all the way to the floor. Or maybe not. Now bring the leg back up and transfer the strap to your left hand. Reach the right hand out to the side and let it land on the floor to provide balance. Now let the right leg move over to the left, but make sure you don't let your right glute lift off the mat. You'll probably notice your leg will move to about a 45-degree angle. With your knee still straight, let your leg move back to the center line of your body and down so that it comes close to the left leg resting on the ground. Then transfer the strap to your right hand again as your right leg sweeps up and over to the right in a big circle. From there see if your leg will continue to sweep up in a big arc with the right foot still on or near the floor and the knee straight (it probably won't). Don't force it. Now release the strap and move to the left side, performing the same motions. What you'll probably notice from this Practice is that the range of motion of the hip joint is greater with your knee bent than when your leg is straight. It's important to notice the difference, but we won't worry about why.

Part 3 – Lie face down on your mat with your legs straight and your feet about hip-width apart. Press the front of both hips into the mat and try not to let them lift up. Bend your right knee to ninety degrees and point your toes on the right foot toward the sky. While still pressing the front of the right hip into the mat, try to lift your right knee up off the mat without arching your back and then return to the starting position. What you probably have found is that your knee wouldn't come up very much at all. Try the Practice again on the left side. One last variation. Keep your right knee straight and try to lift your right foot and knee off the mat while pressing the front of the right side of your pelvis into the mat. Bring your right foot down and try the same thing on the left side. You have probably found that your knee didn't lift up very much, either with the knee bent or straight.

What we've experienced in these Practices is how the hip joint works and specifically how the leg moves around in the hip joint. You can see there's a pretty large range of motion in this joint. The leg can move down and up (at least when the knee is bent) and to both sides and can circle around between those four points. We also found that the leg doesn't move backward very much. This is because the socket of the hip joint faces mostly forward and the motion it allows is therefore focused on the front side of the body. What backward motion you may have experienced was probably the result of arching your back.

Practice 2.3 – The Knee Joint. Part 1 – Move to the wall and turn so the outside of your left shoulder and your left hip are facing the wall. You can steady yourself by resting the back of your left hand against the wall. Stand up nice and tall and then bend your right knee as you lift your right foot off the floor so your right heel lifts up in back of you. Keep your right knee pressing down so it's even with your left knee. Bring your right foot up just to the point where there's a 90-degree angle between the upper and lower parts of your right leg, then see if you can bend the knee even more, lifting the right foot even higher, maybe even bringing the right heel all the way up so it touches your right glute. Now release your foot, straightening the knee and let your right foot come back to the mat for a moment or two. Now lift your right thigh up until it's level with the floor, letting the right knee bend and the right foot dangle as you do that. Once your right thigh is parallel to the floor begin to straighten your right leg and press your right heel away from you, straightening your leg. Release your right leg and let it come down so your leg is straight. Repeat the Practice on the other side after turning to face your right side against the wall.

Part 2 – Keeping your right knee even with your left and with the right foot hanging down and lifted just an inch or so off the floor, see if you can bring your right foot forward without moving your thigh forward. Obviously, you can't because your knee joint doesn't allow movement in that direction. (Note: if you have some slight movement forward at the knee joint, that's called hyperextension. It is normally discouraged in yoga poses and is not good for the joint). Try the same thing, but moving the right foot to the left and to the right. You'll notice what you already know – the knee joint doesn't ordinarily allow movement side to side. Repeat the Practice on the other side.

What you've experienced with this Practice is that the knee joint is essentially a hinge. Unlike the hip joint, which is a ball and socket, the knee permits movement in one direction only. The knee joint doesn't permit side to side movement and it doesn't hinge forward. The only movement you find with your knee is backward hinging. And the range of motion is similarly limited, about 145 degrees. We'll find other hinge joints as we work our way through the Practices. For now, just be aware of the difference in how the hinge joints and ball and socket joints work and the range of motion each permits.

Practice 2.4 – The Ankle Joint. Take a seat on your mat with your legs straight and your spine nice and long. Bend both knees and bring the soles of both feet to the mat with your heels about twelve inches in front of you, keeping the knees about hip-width apart. Lift your right foot off the mat and put your right hand under your right calf and your left hand over your right shin. Press both hands toward one another with the calf and shin sandwiched in between so you can feel the shin muscle and the calf muscle at the same time. Now point the toes on your right foot and press the toes away from you. Now pull the toes toward you as you press your heel away. Repeat a few times and begin to notice that the ankle joint allows your foot to hinge at the bottom of your leg. You can feel the shin and calf muscles engage alternately to facilitate the hinging motion. Allow your foot to return to a neutral position and then begin to move your foot side to side. At first, it may feel like this motion is occurring in the ankle joint. But bring your attention to your knee and you'll notice the side to side motion of the foot occurs from movement in the knee joint and the thigh, not from the ankle joint. You can verify this by pressing your hands on either side of your shin as you move your foot side to side. When you do that you'll notice that it's your lower leg that's pivoting. Complete the Practice by returning your right foot to the mat. Pause for a moment and then repeat the Practice with the left foot and leg. What you experience in this Practice is that the foot hinges forward and back at the ankle joint. Any sideward angular movement is because the leg is rotating in the hip joint, not because the foot is rotating at the ankle.

Practice 2.5 – The Shoulder Joint. Standing on your mat, let both arms dangle at your sides with your palms facing your body. Bring your awareness to your right arm and particularly your shoulder. Keeping your elbow straight, begin to very slowly lift your right arm straight out in front of you until it's parallel to the floor. As your arm lifts, notice how the deltoid muscle engages and imagine the ball at the top of the humerus fluidly rolling in the socket of your shoulder joint. Rotate the palm of your right hand so it's facing up toward the sky and then slowly continue raising your right arm, pressing out through the fingers of the right hand as the arm rises to straight up and overhead. Now reach your fingertips up a little higher, noticing your right shoulder lift toward your right ear as you do that. Then relax your shoulder away from the ear. Do that several times and notice how the back of your shoulder and your shoulder blade rise and fall with the movement. Continue reaching your right arm toward the sky and then, still keeping the right elbow straight, see how far you can without strain bring your right arm to the left toward your head and right ear, but without dropping your left shoulder down or bringing your right shoulder up or forward. Now slowly bring your right arm down toward the floor, again keeping the elbow straight. Once your arm is hanging at your side, continue lifting it up in back of you, keeping both shoulders square to the front. Depending on how flexible you are, your arm may come up as much as 90 degrees from the floor. Take a few moments to explore the movement of the shoulder joint, making sure you keep the elbow straight. Circle your arm around from front to back and side to side and everywhere in between. When you're done exploring and feel like you have a good feeling for the range of motion in the shoulder joint and the way the muscles feel throughout that range of motion, let your right arm drop down by your side. Pause for a moment and then repeat the Practice on the left side.

Practice 2.6 – The Elbow Joint. Stand on your mat facing forward and allow both of your arms to hang down by your sides with the palms facing your body. Keeping the upper part of your arm even with the right side of your body, bend your right elbow and begin to lift your forearm up. As you lift your forearm, see if you can feel what arm muscles you're using to cause the movement. Once the elbow joint is bent to about 90 degrees, slowly let your arm return to its original position. Now rotate your wrist so your palm is facing up and the thumb is pointing out and begin to lift your forearm, bending at the elbow joint. As you do that, bring your attention again to the arm muscles and see if you can now tell which muscles are engaged in the movement. Continue bending past the 90-degree angle we stopped at before and eventually bend your elbow as much as possible, perhaps resting your hand or wrist on your right shoulder. Slowly straighten and bend your arm this way a few times, imagining the elbow joint as a hinge that allows movement up and down only. Also, notice that the elbow joint will not allow the arm to bend beyond 180 degrees. That is, you can't bend backward at the elbow joint. Finally, position your arm so your elbow is bent at 90 degrees and then begin to gently move your right hand out to the side, keeping the right elbow tucked in tightly to the side of your body. Explore that movement a few times, noticing that it's the shoulder joint allowing the outward rotation of the arm, not the elbow joint. Complete the exercise by allowing your arm to fall straight down by your side. Then repeat the exercise on the left side.

Practice 2.7 – The Wrist Joint. Take a comfortable seat on your mat. Lift your right arm, bending at the elbow until the elbow joint is bent to about 90 degrees. With your right-hand open and fingers pointing straight forward, rotate at the wrist until your palm is pointing to the left and your thumb is on top. Now firmly grasp your right wrist with your left hand, pressing your left palm into the inside of the right wrist. Keeping your fingers straight so you don't bend at any of the knuckles, hinge the right hand at the wrist joint and point your fingers off to your left. You'll probably be able to form about a 90-degree angle between your hand and your forearm. Bring your hand back so it's straight and then hinge the other direction at the wrist so the fingers point off to the right. Again, you'll probably find approximately a 90-degree range of motion. Explore the hinging motion of the wrist and imagine the joint as merely a hinge that allows movement side to side, like a door that swings both ways. Now bring your right hand back so its straight and then try to lift the fingers up toward the sky, then back to straight and down toward the mat, making a sort of chopping motion, all the while holding your right wrist with your left hand so the right forearm is immobile. Notice that this is a different type of movement from the side-to-side hinging movement. Now explore the range of motion in the wrist joint by moving your hand through that range of motion. Complete the Practice by releasing the right hand down to your side and then repeat the Practice on the left side.

Practice 2.8 – The Spine – Introduction. You already recognize that the spine is not a single joint, like most of the others we've explored. Instead, it's made up of series of vertebrae stacked one on top of the other. The largest vertebrae are on the bottom and the vertebrae get progressively smaller as you move up toward the head. There are a total of 33 vertebrae, although 9 of them are fused together into the tailbone and the sacrum and don't move independently. The spinal column has five distinct areas, the neck (cervical spine), the thoracic (mid-back), the low back (lumbar), the sacrum (with five fused vertebrae) and the coccyx or tailbone (with four fused vertebrae). The 24 unfused vertebrae interlock and are separated by discs that allow the vertebrae to move independently to some extent. The top vertebra connects directly to the skull and allows for the "yes" motion of the head and the second highest vertebra allows for the side to side "no" motion of the head. For our purposes, think of the whole vertebral column as a complex joint that allows movement in a variety of directions, which we'll now explore.

Practice 2.8 – The Spine – Side Movement. Bring your mat to the wall and place the short end against the wall. Stand with your back to the wall with your feet hip-width apart and your heels a few inches away from the wall. Lightly press your glutes, shoulder blades and the back of your head into the wall. Leave your left arm by your side and reach your right arm up and overhead, extending your fingertips toward the sky. Keep your hips level and reach your right hand over to the left, making sure your right shoulder blade continues to press against the wall. Continue pulling the right hand over further to the left as you feel the top of your spine curving to the left. Come back to center, then drop your right hand down by your side and repeat the Practice on the left side, feeling the top of the spine curve to the right. Return to center and bring both arms down by your sides.

Practice 2.9 – The Spine – Rounding. With the long end of your mat against the wall, stand with your back to the wall as in Practice 2.8. With your tailbone, shoulder blades, the back of your shoulders and the back of your head gently pressing into the wall, bring your right hand behind you and feel the space between the wall and your lumbar spine, the lower part of your back. Notice how the spine curves away from the wall and toward your navel in this area. Bring your hand back down by your side. Continue pressing your tailbone into the wall and begin to round your back, bringing your shoulders and shoulder blades away from the wall and your chin to your chest. Continue rounding as you reach the top of your head down toward your feet and try to keep your forehead as close as possible to your chest. Round down, but no farther than the point where the top of your head is about even with your waist and then pause and notice how your spine has rounded. On an in-breath, slowly rise back to the starting position.

Practice 2.10 – The Spine – Arching. With your mat against the wall as in Practice 2.9, stand facing the wall. Make sure your big toes, pubic bone, chest and forehead are gently resting against the wall. Notice that your body is in the straight shape, with knees over feet, hips over knees, shoulders over hips and your head centered in a neutral position. Now begin to slowly lift your chin toward the sky and away from your chest, allowing your forehead to move away from the wall. As you keep contact between your pubic bone and the wall, begin to arch your back and allow your chest to move away from the wall. If it feels ok, allow your head to drop back even more and look up toward the sky. Continue bending backward only to the point where you can keep contact between your pubic bone and the wall. Once you reach the point where further backward bending will pull your pubic bone away from the wall, pause for a moment and notice the arched shape of your spine – seeing how it's curving backward. On your next inhale, slowly bring your chin back down so it's level and then flatten your back, rising to the starting position, completing the Practice.

Practice 2.11 – The Spine - Twisting. Come to a seat on your mat in any comfortable cross-legged position. Sit up nice and tall. As you breathe in let your spine extend a bit longer and feel the crown of your head rising up toward the sky. Keep your gaze level and try not to lift your chin up. Keeping your spine long, reach both arms out to a T, gently stretching your hands away from one another. Now take a twist to the left, still keeping the spine long, and bring the palm of your right hand down so it rests on the top of your left knee. Bring the left hand down to the mat behind you. Take a deep breath in and lengthen your spine again as you bring your gaze over your left shoulder. Make sure you're pressing down equally on your sitting bones, particularly the right one. Pause and take a couple of breaths, visualizing the vertebrae in your spine twisted to the left. Perhaps you can imagine your spine as a wet dishcloth being wrung out by the twisting action. Take the time to notice the mechanics of the twist. Notice that before you started the twist, your shoulders and hips were in the same plane and after you twisted, the shoulders and hips are in different planes, perhaps as much as 90 degrees apart from one another. This is the essence of the twist. It doesn't involve any rounding or arching of your spine. The spine has remained flat throughout the movement. After you have a good feeling of the twisting motion, release back to the center by reaching both of your arms up and overhead and then back down to your lap, completing the Practice. Pause for a few moments and then repeat the Practice on the other side, twisting to the right.

Congratulations on completing the Practices in this Chapter. I hope they have helped you understand the basic joints in your body, the way each of those joints works and the movements each joint is capable of.

Chapter 3 – Understanding Basic Body Shape

In this Chapter we'll look at three basic body shapes. In every yoga pose you learn you'll be able to identify one of these three basic body shapes. While Block of Clay was most helpful in our explorations in Chapter 2, we need something a little more refined to guide us through Chapters 3, 4 and 5. So I've recruited my dear friend Mr. Yoga to help us. Mr. Yoga has limbs, joints and proportions that are more or less approximately the same as those of a human body.

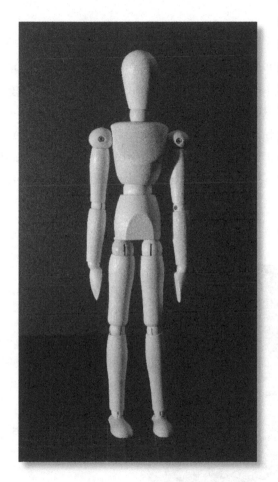

As we saw in Chapter 2, the joints in the human body provide a significant range of motion that allows the body and limbs to be positioned in nearly infinite ways. For example, look at the upright stance shown in the picture to the left. Both arms can be pointing directly down or the arms could be extended up or out or front or back or one arm could be down and the other out or the arms could be down and the head tilted to the left or the right or forward or back. My head is about to explode with the possible variations and we haven't even begun to consider the variations that could be achieved by bending one or both of the elbows or twisting the torso or bending the knees. If you could count each fraction of a degree of change in the positioning of an arm, leg, neck or torso, there are literally thousands upon thousands of variations, just for this basic standing posture. While recognizing this reality, let's not get lost in the potential complexity and, instead, let's simplify and think about the body in a more basic, more macro sort of way. When we do that, we can distill the shape a body can take into just three possibilities: straight, hinged at the hips or curved. We'll examine each of those three shapes in this Chapter.

Straight Body Shape. If you're brand new to yoga, you don't know that Mr. Yoga in the picture on the last page is positioned in a common yoga pose. For the moment, let's not worry about the yoga name for this position, which we'll get to later on. What we can see right away though is that this is an obvious straight body shape. We can define the straight body shape this way: the body is arranged symmetrically from side to side, with the hips aligned over the heels, the shoulders over the hips and the head aligned in a neutral position at the top of the spine.

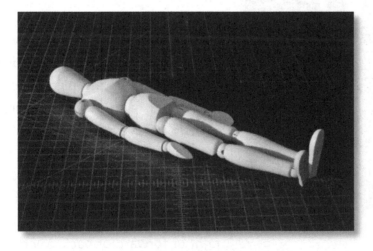

We can also imagine other positions that would have the same basic straight body shape, as shown in the picture to the left, where Mr. Yoga is lying face up.

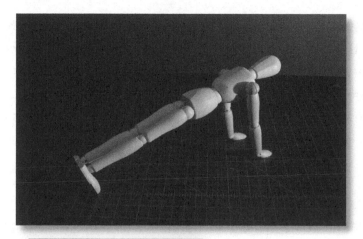

You can see the same shape in the picture a left, where he's doing a plank face down.

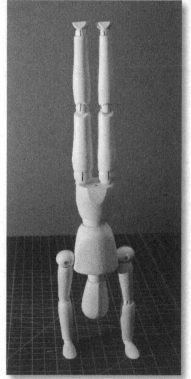

Finally, check out this picture, where Mr. Yoga is upside down, and notice that he's kept the same basic straight body shape. Again, let's not be concerned about whether these are actual yoga poses or not or what they're called. Instead, let's just recognize that in each position, the body is straight, as we've defined the straight body shape.

As the pictures illustrate very clearly, Mr. Yoga's body shape is the same in each of these positions. His heels, knees, hips and shoulders are all aligned and his head is centered in a neutral position on the shoulders. That is of course not to say that the effect on the body is the same in each of the different positions. Obviously, each one would impose very different conditions for the body to deal with, such as what part of the body is bearing weight and so on. For the present, the point to understand is a simple one: Mr. Yoga retains his straight body shape regardless of how his body is differently orientated in space.

Practices

The following Practices will help you begin to understand and feel the straight body shape.

Practice 3.1 – Move to a bare wall and stand with your back to the wall. Place your feet about hip-width apart and make sure your heels are lightly touching the wall. With your knees straight but not hyperextended, gently press the back of your calves, your glutes, your shoulder blades, the back of your shoulders and the back of your head into the wall. Try not to arch your back or lift your chin and let your arms hang loosely by your side. Now close your eyes and just notice what it feels like to have your body aligned in this straight position. Feel the weight distributed evenly between your heels and the balls of your feet. Feel your knees stacked over the front of your ankles and your hips over your knees. Feel your spine rising from your pelvis and your shoulders stacked over your hips. Finally, feel your head resting comfortably at the top of your spine, not bending forward or back or to either side. Take five breaths, still with the eyes closed. When you've completed the breaths, open your eyes and step away from the wall, bringing the Practice to an end.

Practice 3.2 – Move to your mat and lie down on your back in a supine (face up) position. Make sure your legs are straight and your knees aren't bent and have your feet about hip-width apart. Reach away from your hips with your heels and make sure the toes of both of your feet are pointing straight up to the sky. Let your arms be straight and by your sides with your palms facing up. Make sure your elbows are straight. Check in with your chin, making sure it's not lifted up away from your sternum (breastbone) or tucked down toward the sternum. Now close your eyes and feel the back of your heels, your calves, the back of your knees, the back of your thighs, your glutes, your shoulder blades, the back of your shoulders, the back of your arms, your elbows, the back of your hands and the back of your head, all resting gently on the mat. Remember what it felt like when you were standing against the wall in the last Practice. Become aware that the alignment of your body at this moment is the same as it was when you were laying down. Your body is straight. Your knees are aligned with your ankles, your hips are aligned with your knees, your shoulders are in line with your hips and your head is centered between your shoulders. Nothing is bending or twisting. Take five breaths, still with eyes closed, and then slowly open your eyes and come to a seat, completing the Practice.

Practice 3.3 – Fold a heavy blanket into a packet that's about two inches thick and about a foot wide and as long as you need it to be with the blanket you're using. Return to your mat and lie down on your back and put the blanket on your mat so the foot-wide edge is touching your right hip. Reach your right arm straight out to the right and then roll your body over onto its right side. You may need to lift your right hip off the mat and slide the blanket under your hip so the hip rests on the blanket. Bend your right elbow and support your head with your arm or, if it's more comfortable, rest your head on a blanket or block or pillow. Rest your left leg, including the foot, on the inside of your right leg. Rest your left arm on top of your left side, making sure your arm is centered. Press lightly through the heels of both feet, lengthening your legs from your hips. Lengthen the neck, gently pressing the top of your head (the crown) away from your shoulders. Close your eyes. Now feel the alignment of your body. Your knees are in line with your ankles, your hips are lined up with your knees and your shoulders are lined up with your hips. Your head is centered on your shoulders. Nothing is bent or twisted. Your body is straight, just like it was when you were standing against the wall and when you were laying on your back. Take five breaths and then slowly open your eyes, rolling to your back. Come to a seat as you complete the Practice.

Practice 3.4 – If you can hold a plank for ten seconds or so, perform this practice. If not, skip it and do the next one instead. Come down to your mat and lie on your belly. Bring your hands to the mat right under your shoulders and press the palms of both of your hands into the mat. Tuck your toes so the bottom of the toes are pressing down on the mat and press back on your heels. Now stiffen your body and push up to a plank, making sure both arms are straight and your elbows aren't bent. Close your eyes and align your body so it's straight, just like in Practices 3.1, 3.2 and 3.3. Notice that your heels, knees, hips and shoulders are all in a straight line and your back is flat. Your head is centered on your shoulders and isn't twisting left or right. Your neck is in line with the rest of your spine and your chin is neutral, not lifting away from your chest or tucking in toward the chest. Take a few breaths, imagining that as you breathe in you are able to send the breath all the way from your heels, up the back of your legs and then along your spine to the crown of your head and as you exhale the breath follows the same path down the backside of your body. Gently open your eyes, bring your knees to the mat and then lower all the way down, completing the Practice.

Practice 3.5 – If it's too much of a challenge to hold a full plank, there's another way to get the same feeling by performing this Practice instead. Fold a thick blanket in half length-wise so it's about as wide as your mat. Lay the blanket on the mat so the bottom of the blanket is about one-third of the way up from the bottom of the mat. The top of the blanket can extend above the top of the mat. Now lay down on the blanket face down, with your knees just below the bottom of the blanket so your knees rest on the mat, not the blanket. Reach your arms forward and let your palms rest on the blanket like Superman flying. Keep your forehead on the blanket and make sure you don't twist your head to one side or the other. Also check in with your chin and make sure it's not tucked towards your chest or lifted away from your chest. Finally, point your toes and lightly press your toenails and the tops of your feet into the mat. Now close your eyes. Feel the alignment of your body. Notice that your body is straight. Your knees are in line with your heels, your hips are lined up with your knees and your shoulders are lined up with your hips. Your head is centered on your shoulders and nothing is bent or twisted. Your body is straight, just like it was when you were standing and lying on your back and side. Inhale and imagine you are pulling the breath up from your heels along the back of your legs, up your spine and to the crown of your head. As you exhale, send the breath down that same path. Breathe in and out five times, feeling the breath moving in a straight line up and down. Then gently open your eyes, completing the Practice.

Hinged Body Shape. The second shape the body can take is hinged at the hips.

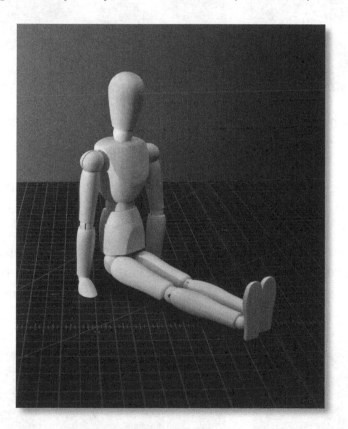

In this position, the body is symmetrical from side to side when it's viewed from the front or the back, but when viewed from the side, the legs and torso form an angle that's less than 180-degrees. To illustrate the concept, let's assume an angle of about 90-degrees, as shown in the picture to the left, while also recognizing that any angle less than 180-degrees and greater than 0-degrees could be termed a hinged body shape. In this hinged shape, Mr. Yoga's head is arranged over his spine, his shoulders are aligned with his hips (that is, his back is straight) and his hips are aligned with his knees and feet, just as in the straight shape. The only change the hinged shape makes from the straight shape is that Mr. Yoga's upper legs have rotated in his hip joints so his legs and his torso form a 90-degree angle when viewed from either side. Otherwise, the alignment is the same as in straight body shape.

Other examples of the body in this hinged shape are demonstrated by Mr. Yoga in the four pictures below. Notice that in each one Mr. Yoga's body is hinged at the

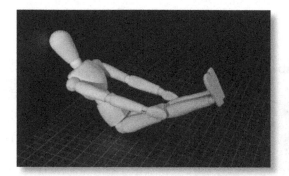 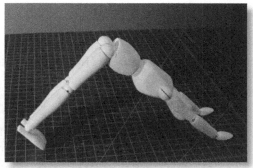

hips at a 90-degree angle, his back is flat, his legs are straight and his torso and neck are straight and not twisted.

In each of these pictures, the basic body shape is the same, with the legs straight, but hinged to a 90-degree angle between the torso and the legs, with the body otherwise aligned as in the straight body shape.

Obviously, each pose presents variations on the basic hinged body shape and the variations arise from differences in how the arms are placed. In two of the situations, the arms are straight and at the sides. In one, the arms are stretched overhead. In another the arms are held straight out and in the last one they are approximately half way between straight out and by the sides.

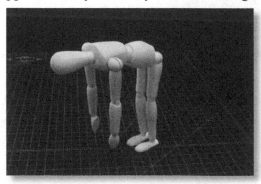 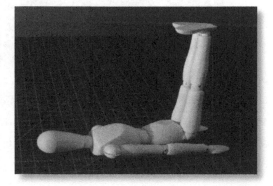

Practices

These Practices will help you begin to feel into the hinged body shape.

Practice 3.6 – Move to the wall and stand with your back to the wall. Repeat Practice 3.1, remembering what it's like to feel your body arranged in a straight line, all the way from your head to your heels. Notice that your back is flat and your shoulder blades, the back of your shoulders and your glutes are pressing lightly against the wall. Now walk your feet forward so your heels are about six inches away from the wall, but keep pressing the glutes gently into the wall. Keep your back flat and your glutes pressing into the wall as you begin to very slowly hinge forward at your hips. Lift your chin just a little bit away from your sternum and reach your forehead forward, helping to keep your back long and straight. Bring the palms of both hands to the top of your thighs. Hinge forward a bit more, keeping your back flat and making sure not to round your shoulders. As you continue to hinge forward at the hips, slowly walk your hands down your legs, making sure you press your palms into your legs instead of grabbing the legs with your fingers. Keep your neck long and in the same line as your spine. Continue hinging forward until your torso forms a 90-degree angle with your legs. Pause when you get there and close your eyes. Feel your straight back. Feel the crown of your head reaching forward, lengthening your neck. Feel your glutes pressing back into the wall. Notice your back is neither rounded nor arched, but is long and straight. Pay particular attention to your low back. If you feel any sense of rounding there, inhale and lift your navel toward your spine. Now take five breaths, moving the breath from your tailbone to the crown of your head with each inhale and sending it back from head to tailbone with each exhale. When you've completed five full breath cycles, allow your back to round deeply and your head to drop down toward your feet. Feel the difference between the flat back and the rounded back. Note: If you feel too much tension in your hamstring muscles as you hinge from standing to the hinged body shape, bend your knees a little. That will allow you to keep your back flat as you come into the shape. Slowly rise back up to standing, completing the Practice.

Practice 3.7 – Move your mat to the wall so the short end of the mat is touching the wall. Come down to the mat and lie on one side with your knees tucked tightly into your chest and your butt touching the wall. Roll over onto your back and straighten your legs. Let your heels rest on the wall with your feet about hip-width apart. Press your sacrum gently into the mat and press your heels up toward the sky. Concentrate on flattening your back. Now close your eyes and breathe slowly and deeply, imagining the breath moving on your inhale from your tailbone to the top of your head and then back on the exhale. On the next inhale allow the breath to move from the tailbone to the heels and then back to the tailbone on the exhale. Repeat that same flow a few more times. Notice your back is straight and notice that your legs are straight. Notice the upper and lower body are hinged at the hips and form about a 90-degree angle. When you're confident that you really feel the shape, let the Practice come to an end and come out of the pose the same way you came in. Note: if you can't straighten your knees with your butt against the wall, move away from the wall a few inches. It's more important to keep the legs straight for this Practice than to achieve exactly a 90-degree angle. So, if the angle is a little less than 90, don't worry about it.

Practice 3.8 – This Practice is similar to 3.7, but is done away from the wall. Lie down on your mat on your back. Repeat Practice 3.2, remembering the feeling of your perfectly straight body. Direct your attention to your glutes pressing into the mat. Then let your attention move up to your shoulder blades and feel them both pressing into the mat. Let your attention rise a little higher and feel the sensation of the back of your shoulders pressing down gently into the mat. Notice that your legs are straight, with your knees not bent. Bring your arms to the mat and by your side with your palms facing down. Continue pressing your entire back from the hips to the back of your head into the mat as you begin to lift both feet off the mat. You can press your palms into the mat to help your legs rise up. Keep your knees straight and continue to lift your feet higher and higher, pressing your heels away from you until your feet are directly over your hips. Now let your eyes close and feel your body hinged at a ninety-degree angle. Feel the flatness of the space from your hips up to your head and from your hips down to your heels. On your next inhale, imagine you are moving the breath from your tailbone up to the crown of your head and as you exhale, send the breath from the top of your head back to your tailbone. On your next inhale, send the breath from your tailbone to the soles of your feet and then inhale the breath back from the heels to the tailbone. Continue for three cycles of breath. When that's complete, bend your knees and bring your feet gently to the mat and open your eyes, completing the Practice. Note: if it's too much of a challenge to lift your feet off the mat with your legs straight, then perform the Practice by bending your knees, bringing them into your chest and then straightening the legs and pressing your heels up toward the sky. If your hamstrings are too tight to allow you to bring your legs straight up, then perform the Practice with your knees deeply bent, letting your heels flop down toward the back of your legs. As you bend your legs at the hips, lift your knees until they point straight up toward the sky. With this variation, instead of pressing up through the heels as you come into the shape, press your knees up to the sky.

Curved Body Shape. The only other basic shape the body can assume is to curve the spine forward, back or to either side. In backward and forward curves, the body is symmetrical on the right and left side when viewed from the front or back, just like it is in the straight body shape. We create a forward curve of the body by beginning with the straight body shape and bending the spine in a forward arc, increasing the spaces between the back of each vertebra and decreasing the spaces in the front. A backward curve is created the opposite way, decreasing the spaces between the back of each vertebra and increasing the spaces in the front.

With side curves, both when curving left and right, the shoulders, hips and feet are no longer symmetrical or aligned when viewed from the front or back. Instead, a side curve (when viewed from front or back) is introduced into the spine. In any of these basic curved body variations, the neck and head naturally follow the curve of the spine, trending forward in forward curving poses, back in backward curving poses and to the left or right in side curves.

The pictures below show four positions that involve forward, back and side bends. As has been true throughout this Chapter, don't worry about whether these are even real yoga poses or what they might be called. We'll get to that before long. Just notice the shapes.

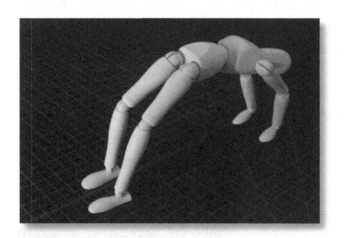
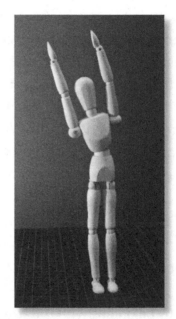
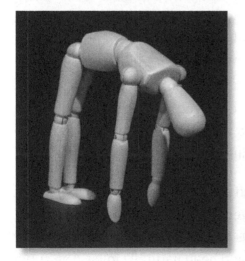
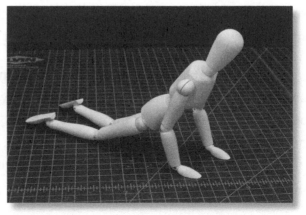

Practices

The following practices will help you begin to feel into and understand the curved body shape.

Practice 3.9 – Lie on your mat face up with your legs straight. Take a moment to settle into the mat and feel your straight body as in Practice 3.2. Now bend both of your knees and hug them tightly into your chest, wrapping your forearms around your knees. Lift your head off the mat and bring your forehead toward your knees and your chin to your chest, curling into a little ball. Let your eyes close softly and bring your awareness to your spine. Imagine the spine all the way from your tailbone to the top of your neck. Feel how your spine curves forward deeply and notice the way your back feels in this rounded position. Become aware that the insides of your shoulders are reaching toward one another. Visualize each individual vertebra and how your shape has brought the top and bottom of the front of each vertebra closer together while the back side of each vertebra has moved farther apart. Breathe in and imagine the breath rising along your back from your tailbone to the back of your head in a long slow arc. As you exhale, send the breath along that same arc and back down to your tailbone. Take a total of five breaths and then release the back of your head gently to the mat. Release your arms from the knees and bring your tailbone back to the mat feeling your back flatten out as you bring the soles of your feet to the mat. Open your eyes as you complete the Practice.

Practice 3.10 – Lie on your mat face down with your legs straight and toes untucked so the tops of your feet are resting on the mat. Feel your body in a straight line from your heels to the crown of your head. Come up to your hands and knees with your hands directly below your shoulders and your knees directly under each hip. Flatten your back by reaching out through the crown of your head and through the tailbone at the same time, lengthening your spine. Now lift your chin away from your chest and at the same time let your belly drop down as you feel a deep arch come into your back. Imagine you're reaching your tailbone away from your knees and allow the arch in your back to deepen. On your next exhale begin to bring your chin toward your chest, press your hands deeply into the mat and round your back. Continue flowing between these two positions, feeling your back arch on the inhale and round on the exhale. Close your eyes and visualize your backbone rounding and arching, bending and flexing, flowing through the Practice five times. Come back to a straight and neutral spine, neither rounded nor arched, and complete the Practice.

Practice 3.11 – Come to hands and knees on your mat, just as you did in the last practice. Walk your hands forward on the mat about nine inches so your hands are well forward of your shoulders. Breathe in deeply as you lift your chin toward the sky and glide your hips forward and down and feel your back begin to arch backward. Straighten your elbows and reach your heart forward, letting your belly drop down. Now let your eyes close and direct your attention to your spine. Feel it arching backward quite deeply. On your next inhale, press a little more deeply into the backbend, but without strain. Don't worry about trying to lift your chin up too much, particularly if you feel tightness in the back of your neck. As you breathe in feel the breath rising along the front of your body from your pubic bone to your throat and as you exhale, send the breath along the same route back to your pubic bone. Take a total of three complete breaths in this way and then bring your chin down so your neck flattens out as you press through both hands so the hips move back toward the heels. Let your hips settle on your heels and stretch your arms forward on the mat, letting your chest come down to the mat at the same time. Feel how your back has flattened as you complete the Practice.

Practice 3.12 – Come to a kneeling position on your mat with your knees slightly more than hip-width apart, padding the knees if you feel uncomfortable in the kneeling position. Reach your arms up and overhead so your upper arms are beside your ears and your elbows are straight. Make sure your hips are directly over your knees and your shoulders are over your hips. Notice that your body is in a straight line all the way from your knees through your outstretched fingertips. Let your left arm drop down loosely by your left side and hang there as you reach the right hand up toward the sky just a little bit more. Now begin to reach the right hand up and over to the left, continuing to reach up as much as you're reaching over. Try not to bring the right hand, elbow or shoulder forward at all; keep everything reaching up and over. Notice the stretch that's coming into your right side-body and feel the stretch from your armpit down to your hip. Soften your effort a little, but keep the same shape and allow your eyes to close. Visualize your spine and imagine it curving to the left. On your next inhale, imagine the breath is rising from your right hip up the right side of your body all the way up and past the armpit and to the fingertips of the right hand. On your exhale, send the breath down the right side of your body to the right hip. Take three long and slow rounds of breath. When you complete the breathing Practice allow your left hand to lift up and meet the right as you begin to straighten your body. Finish by stretching both hands to the sky, feeling the spine lengthen. Keep the spine long as you allow your hips to drop down to your heels and then bring your palms to your thighs. When you're ready, repeat the Practice on the other side.

Practice 3.13 – Move to a bare wall and stand with your back to the wall. Place your feet about hip-width apart with your heels about three inches from the wall. With your knees straight but not hyperextended, gently press your glutes, your shoulder blades, the back of your shoulders and the back of your head into the wall. Try not to arch your back or lift your chin and let your arms hang loosely by your sides. Reach both arms up and overhead and interlace your fingers, pointing the index fingers. Reach the index fingers high, straightening both elbows. Begin bending to the left and let your hips move to the right. Notice the deep side bend in the spine as you keep reaching out through your fingertips. On your next inhale, return to center and then repeat the Practice on the other side, allowing your hips to move left as your fingertips reach up and over to the right. Bend as deeply to the side as you can and then inhale and return to center. Release your arms to your sides as you complete the Practice.

Practice 3.14 – Come back to the wall in the same position as the last Practice. Reach both arms up and overhead and then interlace your fingers and bring your palms to the back of your head with your elbows reaching out and away from one another. Take a deep breath in and as you exhale, while still keeping contact between both shoulder blades and the wall, drop your left elbow down as you reach your right elbow up to the sky. Try not to let your right elbow come forward away from the wall as you bend even more deeply to the left, feeling a deep stretch on the right side of your torso. Visualize your spine bending to the left and coming into a "C" shape. Take a few breaths and come back to center on an exhale. Release your hands and let your arms come down to your sides, completing the Practice. After a couple of breaths, repeat the Practice on the other side, stretching the left side body and visualizing your spine coming into a "C" shape while bending to the right.

Chapter 4 – How is the Body Orientated in Space?

After body shape, the second broad variable we need to explore to understand any yoga pose is how the body is oriented in space when performing the pose; that is, how it is oriented to a hypothetical horizon. We've already seen some of those possibilities in the last Chapter. But now let's approach the question more systematically. Subject to some minor variations, there are just five options for how the body can be oriented in space. They are: upright (standing), inverted (upside down), supine (face up), prone (face down) and on the side.

Straight Shape Orientations

Let's begin with the straight shape we learned about in Chapter 3. It's easy to see that the straight body shape can be oriented in an upright position, inverted,

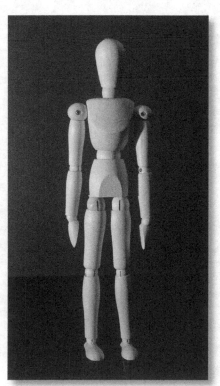

supine, prone and on the side, as illustrated in the picture on this page (upright) and the four pictures on the next page. Notice that in each of the five spatial orientations, Mr. Yoga maintains the straight body shape, with his heels, knees, hips and shoulders all aligned and his head centered on his shoulders. Leaving aside for the time being the variations that result from different positioning of the arms, which we will cover in Chapter 5, the body is in exactly the same shape in each of the five different spatial orientations.

Subject to variations of degree, these are the only ways the straight body can be oriented in space. It isn't a coincidence that each of these different orientations

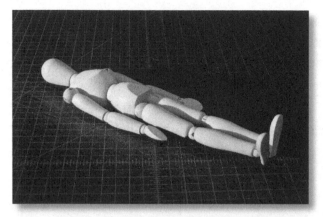

of the straight body shape is a distinct and separately recognized yoga pose. Standing upright is called Mountain Pose, lying face up is called Corpse Pose, face down is called Plank Pose, upside down is called handstand or headstand and the side-oriented posture is called Side Plank Pose.

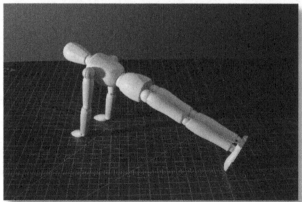

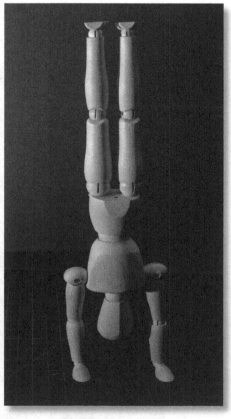

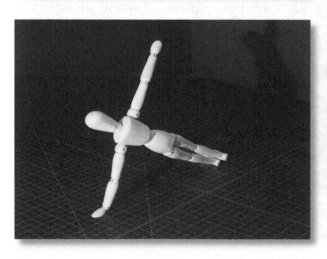

Practices

Practice 4.1 – Stand on your mat in the basic upright straight body shape. Allow your eyes to gently close and feel your knees stacked over your ankles, your hips over your knees, your shoulders over your hips, your spine long and your head centered between your shoulders. Let your arms rest by your sides with your hands in a comfortable position. Notice that your weight is distributed evenly between your left and right foot and between the toes and the heel of both of your feet. Form a distinct mental impression of the straight body shape and hold that in your mind as you come down to your mat and lie on your back, finding that straight body shape again. Close your eyes and reinforce the mental impression of the straight body shape, noticing this time that you're lying on your back.

Practice 4.2 – Continuing from Practice 4.1, roll over onto your belly, untuck your toes (so your toenails are pressing on the mat), let your arms rest by your sides and your forehead rest gently on the mat. Notice that you have retained the straight body shape, although this time your body is oriented face down. With your eyes still closed, tuck your toes, bring your hands under your shoulders, stiffen your whole body and press your palms into the mat, pressing up to a plank. Try to maintain the straight body shape with your heels, hips, shoulders and head all in a straight line. If you can do it without strain, maintain this posture for a few moments and feel the straight body shape. If you have someone who can assist you, ask them to confirm that your hips are level with your heels and shoulders. If they aren't, then adjust the level of the hips until the straight body shape is achieved. Breathe in and out a few times and recognize that your body is in the same straight body shape as before, but now oriented so you're facing down. Release your knees to the mat and take a few breaths.

Practice 4.3 – Continuing from Practice 4.2, bend your left elbow and roll over to your side, making sure the left elbow is directly below your left shoulder. Stack your right foot on top of your left foot. Now press the heels of both feet away from you and use your core to lift your left hip off the mat until there's a straight line between the outside of your left foot, your left hip and your left armpit. Lengthen through the top of your head, taking care that your head is centered on your shoulders, that your gaze is level and that your neck and head are in a straight line with your spine. If available, have someone verify your body is in the straight shape and adjust as needed. With your eyes closed, feel the straight body pose and take a few breathes, noticing that you are oriented on your side. When you're confident in the feeling of the pose, release your left hip to the mat, roll to the other side and repeat the Practice on the right side.

Practice 4.4 (Optional) – If you feel very confident in your ability to perform a handstand against the wall and hold it for a few breaths, you can proceed with this Practice. If you've never done a handstand, haven't done one in a long time or don't know if you can do one, then please skip this Practice for now. Please use a spotter for this Practice. Begin with the short end of your mat against the wall. Facing the wall, bring your hands down to the mat about a foot from the wall, about shoulder width apart, with the thumbs facing one another and the fingers spread wide. Let your head hang down and slowly walk your feet toward your hands and allow your shoulders to move forward of your hands so your shoulders are closer to the wall than your hands are. When your hips are directly over your hands, allow one and then the other leg to float up until your heels gently touch the wall. Now press up through the balls of both feet, lengthening all the way from the shoulders to feet. Notice if you have arched your back. If you have, hug your navel to your spine and flatten your back while continuing to press up through your feet. Take a breath and bring back to mind the feeling of the straight body shape in the standing, prone, supine and side orientations. Then notice that this is the same shape, only in the inverted orientation. After a couple more breaths, release your feet slowly to the mat, then bend your knees and remain in a kneeling position for a few moments to allow the blood pressure to equalize. When you feel ready, rise to complete the Practice.

Hinged Body Shape Orientations

When we move on to the hinged body shape, we find a few different possible options: upright standing, upright seated, prone, supine, inverted and sideways.

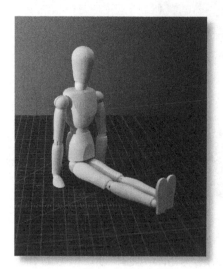

Again, it isn't a coincidence that each of these different orientations of the hinged body shape is a commonly performed and recognized yoga pose. Staff Pose, shown in the picture to the left, is the hinged shape seated. Standing Half Forward Fold, pictured below, is the shape done upright.

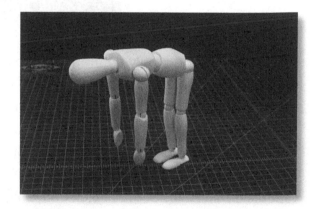

Downward Facing Dog, below left, is the shape in the prone (face down) orientation. Boat Pose, below right, is the hinged shape orientated supine (face up).

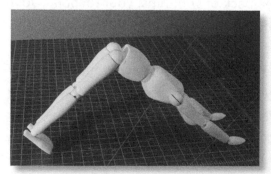
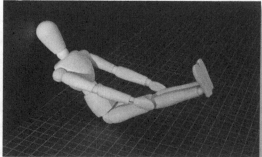

Finally, Legs Up the Wall Pose, modeled by Mr. Yoga in the picture below, is another supine orientation of the hinged shape.

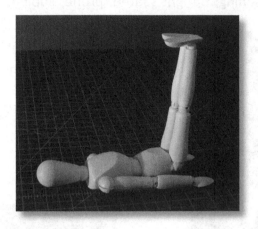

Notice that the only difference in the basic shape of these five different body configurations, other than orientation to the horizon, is arm position. In the first and last pictures, Mr. Yoga's arms are at his sides. In the second picture his arms are stretched forward relative to his torso. In the third picture they are overhead. And in the fourth picture his arms are halfway between at the sides and stretched out. Notice particularly that Mr. Yoga's back is flat in each of the five different spatial orientations of the hinged body shape.

Practices

Practice 4.5 – Bring the short end of your mat to the wall and then sit down facing away from the wall. Gently press the back of your hips, your tailbone, your shoulder blades and the back of your head against the wall as you sit up nice and tall. Bring your hands down to the mat just outside your hips and press your palms into the mat as you take a deep breath in, elongating your spine without lifting your chin. As you press your heels away from you feel the flatness of your lower body all the way from the hips to the heels. Now shift your attention to your upper body and feel the straightness of your upper body all the way from the sitting bones pressing into the mat to the crown of your head reaching toward the sky. Breathe in and imagine the breath rising from your tailbone to the top of your head. Breathe out and imagine the breath traveling down the spine to the tailbone. On your next inhale, imagine the breath traveling from your tailbone to your heels and on your in-breath, imagine the breath retracing that path and coming back to the tailbone. Repeat the breathing Practice a few times, lengthening from the pivot point at the hips each time. Complete the Practice by returning to a normal breath.

Practice 4.6 – Stand near the wall facing away from it. Bring your heels about six inches from the wall and allow your hips to be directly over your feet so your butt is not resting against the wall. Allow your shoulders to align over your hips. Now close your eyes for a moment and recognize your classic standing straight body shape. Keep your upper body straight and try not to bend your knees as you hinge at the hips and bend forward. Let your butt move back and press gently against the wall and as you pivot down, begin to walk your hands down your legs using your arms to support the upper body. Continue hinging at the hips until your upper and lower bodies form a 90-degree angle. Now reach out through the top of your head and lift your heart a bit to lengthen your spine. It may also help to very slightly lift your chin away from your chest. Pause for a moment and recognize the hinged body shape, this time oriented in a standing position. With eyes closed, imagine that you could inhale from the soles of your feet to your tailbone and then exhale from your tailbone to the crown of your head. After trying a few rounds of breath that way, on your next inhale, slowly rise back up, avoiding any rounding in the back and emphasizing the hinging of the upper and lower bodies at your hips. Complete the Practice by returning to the straight body shape.

Practice 4.7 – Come down to hands and knees on your mat. Make sure your hands are right under your shoulders, that they're about shoulder width apart and that your knees are under your hips. Remember the feeling of the hinged body shape as tuck your toes, bring your knees off the mat, begin to straighten your legs and press your hands away from your hips, flattening out your back. Take a moment to notice any rounding of your back and do your best to flatten it out, just like we did in Practices 4.5 and 4.6. If you feel like your back is rounding, press your hands into the mat and at the same time press your tailbone up and back and try bending your knees just a little. Let your head either drop down or keep your ears even with your biceps. Try to avoid lifting your chin away from your chest as that will cause you to arch your back. Close your eyes and imagine that you can send the breath from the palms of your hands to your tailbone and then from your tailbone to your feet. Then lift the breath from the feet to the tailbone and then from the tailbone to the hands. Repeat the breath Practice a few times. When completed, bend your knees and bring them to the mat and remain kneeling for a moment or two before you end the Practice.

Curved Body Shape Orientations

Moving on to the third basic shape, curved, we find that it presents the same familiar orientation options and some interesting additional variations. We can see the curved body shape upright, curving forward, back and to the side. We can also imagine the curved body shape upside down, curving forward, back and to the side. Similarly, we can also imagine the curved body shape facing up and facing down, curving forward, back and to the side. Last, we can imagine the curved shape oriented on the side, with the spine curving forward, back and to the side. Following are some examples.

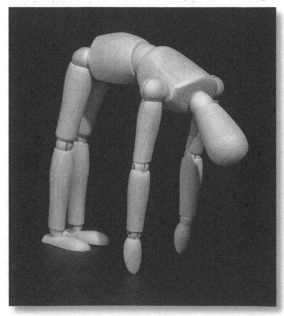

In the picture at left Mr. Yoga is curving forward and rounding his back. Notice he's in the upright orientation.

In the picture below at left he's curving backward (arching). In the example below on the right he's curving to the side in the upright orientation.

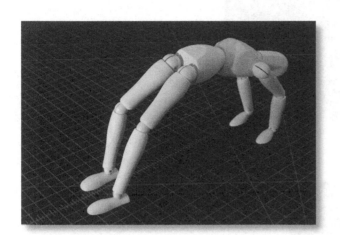

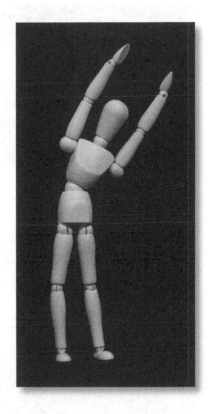

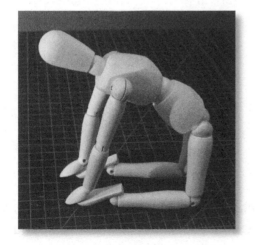

In the picture to the left, you can see the curved body shape in the face-up orientation with the body curving backward.

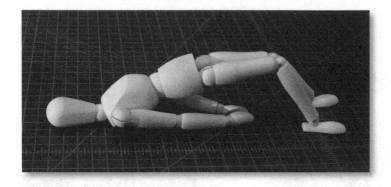

And to the left is another curved body shape, curving backward in the face-up orientation.

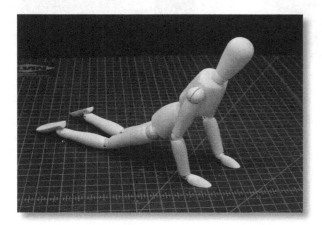

Finally, in the picture at left you can see the curved body shape with the back curving backward (arching) in the face-down orientation.

Practices

Practice 4.8 – Rounded Spine. Take a seat on your mat and bend your knees, bringing the soles of your feet together and allowing your knees to move apart and drop down toward the mat. Bring your chin to your chest and feel your back rounding as you gently allow your forehead to reach down toward your feet. Notice that your spine has rounded all the way from your tailbone to the base of your skull.

As you breathe in, allow the breath to rise up the spine from your tailbone to the back of your head. When you exhale, send the breath back down the rounded spine to your tailbone. Repeat several times, becoming aware of the rounded spine and then slowly release back to the starting position to complete this first phase of the Practice.

Next, lay down on your back and bend your knees, hugging them in tightly to your chest. Lift the back of your head off the mat and bring your forehead toward your knees, touching the knees with your forehead if you can. At the same time, lift your tailbone off the mat, hugging your tailbone toward your chin. Notice that the shape of your spine in this orientation is the same as the first part of the Practice when you were seated. Use the same breath Practice as you did in the first stage and repeat several times. When complete, bring your tailbone and back of your head to the mat, ending the second phase of this Practice.

Finally, bring yourself to a squatting position on the mat with your feet parallel and a little less than hip-width apart. Squat as low down as you can and see if you can keep your heels grounded on the mat as well as the balls of your feet. Not everyone can do that; so don't worry if your heels lift off the mat. Wrap your arms around your legs just below the knees and let your chin come down to your chest. Feel the rounding of your back, just as in phases 1 and 2 of this Practice. After a few moments, release down to a seat and reflect on the fact that the shape of your body in each of the three phases of this Practice was the same. The only difference was that the orientation of the body differed. In phase one, the body was seated. In phase two it was oriented on the back. And in phase three it was upright.

Practice 4.9 – Arched Spine. Begin with your mat against the wall and stand with your heels about 14 inches from the wall with your feet parallel and about hip distance apart. Reach both of your arms up and overhead toward the sky and then begin to lift your chin away from your chest, lifting your gaze upward. Continue reaching up and behind you until both hands touch the wall above and behind your head. Now lift your chest and press your hips forward as you feel a strong arch develop in your spine. Inhale strongly and imagine the breath rising from your navel up to your throat. As you exhale, send the breath back down to the navel. Repeat twice more, noticing that the breath is following the arc of your spine and then bring the Practice to an end by coming back to a standing position.

For phase two of this Practice lie face down on your mat and bring your hands under your shoulders. With your toes untucked, press your palms into the mat and lift your head, shoulders and chest off the mat as you press the tops of your toes and your pubic bone into the mat. Pause for a moment and begin to breathe as in phase 1 of this Practice, imaging the breath moving between the navel and the forehead, following the arc of the spine. Repeat a few times and then end the Practice by lowering back down to the mat.

For the third phase of this Practice, roll over onto your back and bend your knees, keeping the soles of your feet on the mat with your heels right under your knees and your knees not more than hip-width apart. With your arms long and by your sides, press your feet into the mat and lift your hips. Notice the arch in your back and recognize it as the same shape as in phases 1 and 2 of this Practice. The difference is that in the first phase, your body was oriented upright. In the second phase your body was prone (face down) and in the third phase your body was supine (face up). Same shape; different body orientations in space. Bring the Practice to an end by lowering your hips to the mat.

Practice 4.10 – Spinal Side Curve. Begin standing with your back to the wall with your heels a few inches from the wall and your glutes, shoulder blades and the back of your head resting gently against the wall. Now reach your arms up and overhead with the arms straight and bring the palms together and interlace your fingers, except for the index fingers, which you can bring together, pointing straight up. Make sure the backs of both thumbs are gently pressing into the wall. Ground into both feet so you feel stable and solid and then begin to slide your hips to the right while at the same time sliding your interlaced hands to the left along the wall, making sure to keep both elbows straight. Inhale and imagine you can slide the breath up from your right hip to your right armpit and as you exhale, send the breath down from the armpit to the hip, feeling your spine curving to the left. Enjoy three breaths and then bring your hands back to center and try the same Practice on the other side. When you're done, come back to center and release your hands to your sides, completing the Practice.

For phase 2, lie down on your mat, face up. Point your toes and reach your arms up and overhead, like you're doing a full body stretch. Bring your hands together and interlace your fingers, pointing your index fingers, just like in the last phase of this Practice. Feeling your heels, glutes, shoulder blades, the back of your head and your hands in contact with your mat, begin to slide your hands and both feet to the right, keeping the feet together. Keep your arms and legs straight as you do that and feel a distinctive curve, like a crescent moon, in your whole body. Imagine as you inhale your breath is flowing all the way from the inside of the right foot upward along the inside of your body to your hips and then the right armpit and finally to the tips of your index fingers. As you exhale, send the breath back down along that same route to the foot. Do that twice more, noticing the same curved body shape as in the first phase of this Practice, but oriented face up on the mat instead of upright. Now end the Practice, bringing everything back to the starting point. Then do the same thing on the other side.

Let's summarize what we learned from the discussion and Practices in this Chapter. The second variable in yoga poses is how the body is oriented in space. We have seen the body's three basic shapes, straight, hinged at the hips and curved, can be placed in various spatial orientations, including upright, inverted, prone, supine and on the side. Once we know the body shape in the pose and the spatial orientation, we have a lot of information about how to perform the pose. All that remains is to know how the arms, legs, hands, feet, neck and torso are positioned, bent or twisted and we will turn to that next in Chapter 5.

Chapter 5 - Joint and Twisting Variations

In Chapter 3 we considered the overall shape of the body and considered whether it was straight, hinged at the hips or curved. In Chapter 4 we explored how the body was oriented in space. The only thing left to consider before we can completely describe a yoga pose is how the arms and legs are positioned and whether the torso or neck are twisted or not. In this Chapter, we'll examine those variables.

Arms

As we saw and experienced in Chapter 2, the shoulder joint allows your arm to move in a broad range of motion. Your arm can reach straight up, straightforward,

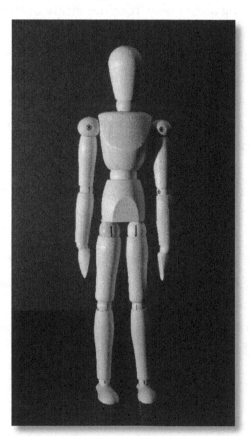

straight down and even straight back. It can also reach straight out to the side and can reach almost everywhere in between. There are of course not regularly practiced yoga poses that use every possible arm position in every possible body position and every possible spatial orientation. However, we can consider some examples of how a change in only the arm position leads to a different pose. In the first example at left, we have the standard straight body shape oriented in the upright position. Notice that Mr. Yoga's arms are both hanging by his sides.

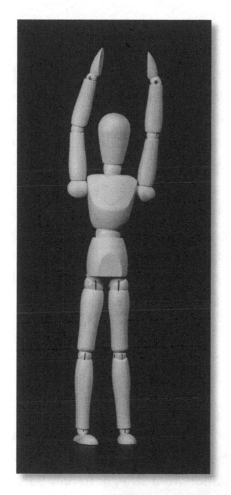

Looking at the picture to the left, you can see the exact same body shape and orientation as in the picture on the prior page (straight body oriented upright), but now the arms are both reaching up and overhead.

Again, notice that the only difference between the two poses is how the arms are positioned. This change in arm position creates a new yoga pose.

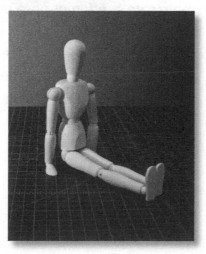

Let's look at another example. In this picture, Mr. Yoga is arranged in the hinged body shape and his orientation is seated upright. Notice his arms are by his sides.

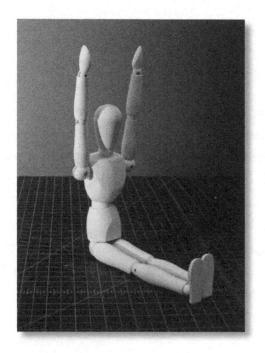

If we raise Mr. Yoga's arms up and overhead, as shown to the left, we've created a whole new pose. Notice again that the only difference between this pose and the one in the last picture is the position of the arms. So you can see that for any particular combination of body shape and spatial orientation, a change in the way the arms are positioned from the shoulder joint will create a different pose.

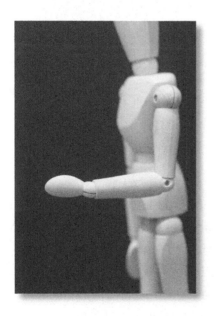

In addition to the shoulder joint, we need to consider the second arm joint – the elbow. As a hinge joint, the elbow moves through about a 140-degree range of motion from straight to fully bent. So, we can create a different pose by bending the arm at the elbow. An example is shown in the picture at left. Here Mr. Yoga is in the straight body shape and is oriented upright. The only change we've made is that his elbow is bent to form a 90-degree angle.

So far we've assumed both arms are doing the same thing at the same time. While that kind of bilateral symmetry in the arm positions is found in many poses,

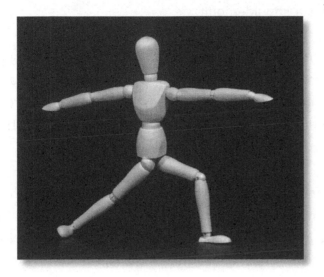

that isn't always the case. In the common pose pictured at left, Mr. Yoga's right arm is reaching forward and his left arm is reaching back. So sometimes the arms aren't symmetrical, but are doing different things. That means we need to consider whether the arm positioning is symmetrical or not.

Let's sum up: as far as the arms are concerned, all we need to look at is how each arm is positioned in the shoulder joint and whether and how the elbows are bent.

Practices

Practice 5.1 – Lie down on your back on your mat and stretch out long, with your arms by your sides. Notice that you are in the straight body shape oriented face up. Bring your awareness to your arms and notice your elbows are straight, your arms are by your sides and your fingers are reaching down toward your feet. As you breathe in keep your arms straight and reach your hands up toward the sky, trying not to lift the back of your shoulders off the mat. As you exhale, notice that the only thing that's happened is that you've pivoted your arms in your shoulder joints.

Practice 5.2 – Continuing from where we left off in Practice 5.1, take another deep breath and reach your arms up and overhead, keeping your elbows straight and allowing the back of your hands to come down and rest on the floor behind you. Take a few breaths as you notice again that you're in the same body shape and orientation as in Practice 5.1 and the only change you've made is that your arms have pivoted further at your shoulder joint.

Practice 5.3 – Continuing from the last Practice, on your next inhale bring your right hand to your left elbow and your left hand to your right elbow and press your elbows behind you while keeping both of your elbows resting on the floor. Breathe in and out a few times and notice the pose is the same as in Practice 5.2, with the exception that both elbows are now bent at 90 degrees.

Practice 5.4 – Continuing from the last Practice, let go of your elbows with your hands and straighten your arms and reach both hands up toward the sky. Then bring your right hand down by your side, leaving your left hand reaching up. Notice that both elbows are straight and unbent, but that the shape is not bilaterally symmetrical. Allow your left arm to come back down by your side, completing the Practice.

Legs

The situation with the legs is similar to the arms. There are two joints to consider that provide a range of movement and positioning possibilities. The hip joint, like the shoulder joint, is a ball and socket joint. The typical range of motion for hip flexion (bringing the thigh up toward the chest) is about 120 degrees. Typical hip extension (bringing the leg backward) is roughly 15 to 30 degrees. Side-to-side motion of the leg at the hip is roughly 40 to 45 degrees out to the side and 20 to 25 degrees inward. The hip joint is also normally capable of about 45 degrees of internal and external rotation. In a yoga pose, we might find the legs in line with the spine, like our classic standing straight body shape, or bent 90-degrees at the hip like in our classic seated hinged body shape.

The other leg joint to consider is the knee. As a hinge joint like the elbow, it bends backward about 150-degrees, but not forward at all. Both knees can be straight or they might both be bent. Also, the legs don't have to be positioned the same on the left and right sides. As is the case with the arms, the legs can also be asymmetrical, multiplying the variations significantly.

Practices

Practice 5.5 - Lie down on your back on your mat. Keeping your knees straight, begin to lift both heels off the mat until your feet are directly above your hips and you've assumed the classic hinged at the hips shape. Press through your heels and at the same time press your sacrum into the mat, making sure your back is flat and you're not lifting your tailbone off the mat.

Practice 5.6 – Begin by standing in the middle of your mat facing the mat's long edge. Step your right foot out to the right about eighteen inches and your left foot out to the left the same distance. Make sure your feet are still parallel and the toes on both feet are facing the same direction as your gaze – toward the long edge of the mat. Now pivot a little on the balls of both feet and bring your heels a little farther apart than your toes. Keeping your spine long and reaching your ears away from your tailbone, reach both arms out to a "T." Next, bending at the hips and not the waist, hinge forward and bring your torso down until it's parallel to the floor. Then bring your hands down so they're pressing into the floor directly below your face. Lengthen your spine, reinforcing the feeling of a flat back, and then notice that your legs are about 45-degrees out to each side and that you're in a hinged body shape with your legs bent about 90-degrees to your torso. After taking a couple of breaths in this shape, bring your hands to your hips, rise back up with a flat back and then step your feet together, coming back to where we began this Practice.

Practice 5.7 – Standing in the middle of your mat and facing the short edge, assume the straight body shape that you already know quite well. Keep the straight body shape from your hips to the top of your head as you begin to bend both knees just a little, allowing your hips to move down and back toward your heels and keeping your knees about hip-width apart. Keep your upper body perpendicular to your mat and try not to hinge forward at your hips. Just a little bend in the knees is enough. Now notice that both your upper legs have moved in your hip joints and the angle between your thighs and your torso has become less than 180-degrees. Also, notice that both knees have bent so the angle between the back of your thighs and the back of your lower legs has become less than 180-degrees. After a few breaths, begin to straighten your legs and come back to where you started.

Practice 5.8 – Stand at the front of your mat facing the short edge. Keep your back as flat as you can and hinge at your hips, bringing your hands down just in front of your feet. If your hands don't reach all the way to the mat, bend your knees as much as you need to so you can press your palms into the mat, taking care to keep your back flat. Now step your left foot back, tuck the toes and bring the left foot to the mat. If you stepped back far enough your right knee should be bent to about a 90-degree angle. Keep your left leg straight and press back on your left heel. Keeping pressing both hands into the mat and reach your ears away from your shoulders, lengthening your neck. Notice that you're in the classic straight body shape, oriented face down, but that your right leg is hinged at the hip and your right knee is probably pressing into your chest. Also notice that your right knee is bent, forming about a 90-degree angle between your upper and lower leg. Finally, notice that the leg positions are not symmetrical. After a few breaths, step your left foot forward until it meets your right foot and then rise back up to your original starting position. Then repeat the Practice on the other side.

Twists

Finally, let's look at twists to complete our exploration of the variables to be considered. In most of the situations we've looked at so far, the torso and neck weren't twisted. However, you will frequently find that a yoga pose takes advantage of the body's ability to twist and this gives us many additional possibilities for each of the straight, hinged at the hips and curved body shapes. The twists we are concerned with are mainly to the torso and to the neck. In some poses both the neck and torso are twisted (sometimes in the same direction and sometimes in the opposite direction). In others, only one or the other is twisted. The spine allows the torso to twist left or right about 90 degrees, more or less.

Notice what twisting means: If we draw a line between the left and right shoulder and another line between the right and left hips, the two lines are parallel when the torso isn't twisted. However, when the torso twists, the shoulders and hips move out of alignment and rotate so that they end up to the point where the line the shoulders are in is about perpendicular (90-degrees apart) to the plane the hips are in. In the picture to the left, Mr. Yoga isn't quite able to twist that much.

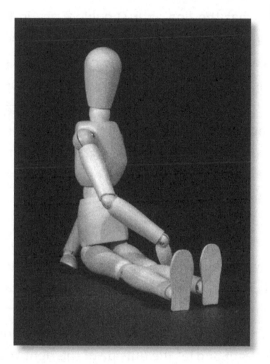

Instead, notice that the planes his shoulders and hips are in are about 45-degrees apart from one another.

The neck has a greater range of motion than the spine. There are two specialized vertebrae that connect the head to the rest of the spine. The top one is called Atlas and it's because of Atlas that you can nod your head "yes." It allows the chin to lift up and away from the sternum and to drop down toward the sternum. The second vertebra that atlas rests on allows atlas to pivot and this joint is responsible for the side to side "no" motion of the head. The head can pivot about 90 degrees side to side for a total twisting movement of about 180-degrees. There are many yoga poses that incorporate the "yes" and "no" and pivoting motions of the neck.

Practices

Practice 5.9 – Sit on your mat with your legs comfortably crossed and one foot in front of the opposite ankle. Feel your sitting bones firmly grounded on the mat. As you inhale feel your spine lengthen and allow your ears to move away from your shoulders. Keep your back nice and flat, not rounding or arching. Now lift your arms out to a "T" and then twist to the left, keeping your spine long as you twist.

Bring your left hand down behind you on your mat, with your hand as close to your butt as you can. Then bring your right palm to your left knee. Breath in deeply and as you exhale twist your upper body to the left. Although you'll be tempted to twist your head the same direction, resist that for a moment and keep your gaze centered so you're looking forward and your head isn't rotating relative to your shoulders. Pause for a moment and take a couple of breaths,

Notice that your spine is twisted so that the line your shoulders are in has rotated relative to the line your hips are in. Now twist your head to the left so you can gaze over your left shoulder and notice that both your torso and your neck have twisted away from center and are twisting the same direction. Keeping your torso twisted to the left, keep your chin level as you twist your neck and bring your gaze over to the right and stare over your right shoulder. Notice now that your neck is twisted in the opposite direction from your torso. Bring your head back to center, taking the twist out of your neck, and then untwist your torso. Take a few breathes and then do the Practice again on the other side.

Practice 5.10 – Lie down on your mat on your back in the straight body shape. Now bend your knees and hug them into your chest. Try not to lift your tailbone or shoulder blades off the mat. Instead, flatten your back, even if that means loosening your grip on your knees. Then release your hands and bring them out to a "T" with your hands outstretched and your palms facing down. Keeping both knees together, allow them to float to the right and let the outside of the right knee land on the floor beside you. Soften your left shoulder, allowing the back of the shoulder to settle into the mat. Keep your gaze up toward the sky. Notice that your left hip is lifted up off the mat and that the plane your hips are in has rotated about 90-degrees from the plane your shoulders are in. Take a couple of breaths as you feel the spinal twist. When you're ready, turn your head to the left, keeping your chin in a neutral position. Now notice that your gaze is about 180-degrees apart from the direction your knees are pointing and that both your torso and your neck are twisted. When you're ready, bring your head back to center and let your knees float back to center. Go ahead and complete the Practice by twisting to the other side. When you've completed both sides, bring your knees back to center and hug them in tightly again, eventually straightening your legs and returning to the straight body shape.

Practice 5.11 – Stand at the front of your mat facing the short edge in the straight body shape. Fold all the way down with a flat back and bring your hands down to the mat on either side of your feet. Pick up your left foot and step it way back so your right knee bends to 90-degrees. Then bring your Knee to the mat behind you and lift your arms up and overhead so your hands are directly above your shoulders and your shoulders are right over your hips. Try not to arch your back. Now bring your arms out to a "T" and reach your hands apart from one another. Twist your torso to the right so your left hand is reaching forward and the right is reaching back and your arms are about 180-degrees from one another. Pause for a moment and take a breath or two as you notice your torso is twisted and your shoulders are rotated about 90-degrees from your hips. Now turn your head so you're gazing toward the sky and notice your neck has now twisted as well as your torso. Bend your left elbow and bring it to the top of your right knee and bend your right elbow and then bring your palms together. Notice that the more you lift your right elbow up the deeper your twist becomes. After a couple of breaths, come out of the twist, bring your hands to the mat on either side of your right foot and step your left foot forward to meet your right, coming back to a standing forward fold. Slowly rise up out of the forward fold to standing. When you're ready, perform the Practice on the other side.

Chapter 6 – Time to Learn Some Poses

Congratulations on all your hard work so far. You've learned a lot about what your body is capable of and how it can move, including:

- The basic shapes your body can assume – straight, hinged at the hips and curved.
- That you can orient each body shape in space in five different ways – upright, inverted, supine, prone and on the side.
- That the basic body shapes can be modified by positioning the arms and legs in different ways and twisting the torso and neck.

I suspect you've also learned even more than you realize. You've learned and your body has experienced all the variables that go into making any yoga pose. So now it's time to bring all of this together and explore some common yoga poses in detail and to begin using the names of the poses that you'll hear in yoga classes. We aren't going to try to learn every yoga pose there is. Instead, we'll stick to the basic ones that you'll be likely to run into in many yoga classes you take. There are three sections in this Chapter. The first section will take you through yoga poses that are based on the straight body shape you've learned. The second section will introduce poses based on the hinged at the hips shape. And the final section will let you learn yoga poses based on the curved body shapes.

Section 1 – Straight Body Poses

In this section we'll learn thirteen common yoga poses that you'll encounter in many yoga classes. Each of these poses is based on the straight body shape.

Mountain Pose *(Tadasana)*

Mountain Pose, or Tadasana as it's called in Sanskrit, is our classic straight body shape oriented upright or standing. The arms, legs, neck and torso are all straight and not bent or twisted. If you look back at Practice 3.1, you'll see it was Mountain

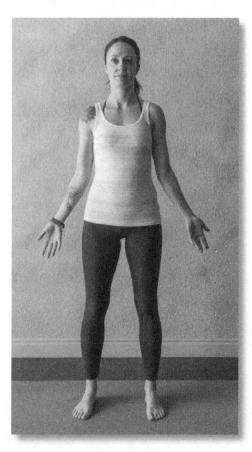

Pose you were experiencing. To move into the pose, stand on your mat with feet parallel and about hip-width apart and the weight distributed evenly side to side and front to back on both feet. In other words, press into the ball of each foot as much as the heels. Let your arms hang down by your sides and rotate your palms so they face forward with the thumbs pointing out. Let your eyes close gently and take a deep breath, feeling your spine lengthen as the crown of your head naturally rises toward the sky. Keep that length in your spine as you breathe out. Imagine your knees stacked over your ankles, your hips over your knees, your shoulders stacked over your hips and your head centered on your shoulders, with your chin level and your gaze straight ahead. If you feel like your low back, the lumbar spine, is arching then bring your navel to your spine and that will take a bit of that arch out of your low back. Remember this is a straight body shape, not a curved shape. With your eyes still closed, enjoy at least five complete rounds of breath before you come out of the pose. If you are unsure about your alignment in Tadasana, repeat Practice 3.1, using the wall to help your body remember the alignment.

Variations: Extended Mountain Pose (Urdhva Hastasana). Start in regular Mountain Pose and then reach your arms up and overhead with your elbows straight, keeping your biceps on either side of your ears as you stretch your

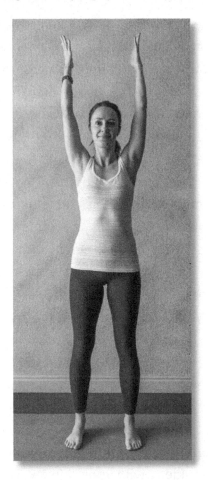

fingertips toward the sky. If your shoulders are tight, you may be tempted to lift your heart too much and begin to arch your back. Resist that temptation, remembering this is a straight body pose, not a curved shape. Avoid arching by not reaching the arms up quite as high and by bringing your navel toward your spine.

Chair Pose *(Utkatasana)*

Chair is a very common pose and you'll probably do it in every yoga class you take. I teach it as a straight body pose that looks like the picture on this page. Notice the back is flat (except for the normal curves of the spine) all the way from the hips through the shoulders and to the top of the head and the arms are

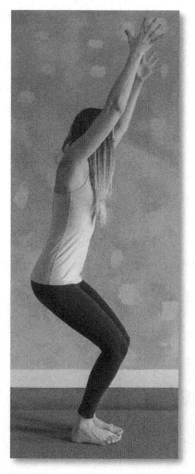

stretched upward in the same line. See how the body is straight from the hips through the fingertips and the upper body is nearly perpendicular to the mat. All we've done to move into chair pose from Mountain pose is to bend both knees, keeping the weight in the heels so the knees don't come too far forward over the toes.

Let's practice Chair Pose. Stand on your mat in Mountain Pose and then lift your arms up and overhead, moving into Extended Mountain Pose. Bring your weight into your heels. Continue to reach up through your fingertips and begin to bend your knees just a bit, bringing your hips down in back of you. There are three things to watch for in the pose. First, remember this is a straight body pose and although there's some hinging at the hips that occurs because your knees are bending, the hip hinging shouldn't come anywhere close to 90 degrees.

In the picture, it's about 45-degrees. Second, avoid bending forward at the waist which would bring your upper body so it's moving toward parallel to the mat. Keep your upper body perpendicular to the mat. Third, try to avoid arching your lower back, the lumbar spine, and instead keep pressing your tailbone down toward your heels, bringing length to your back body.

Corpse Pose *(Savasana)*

Nearly every yoga practice will include Corpse Pose (Savasana) as the final pose of the practice. I had one teacher who would direct students into Savasana and then tell them: "Enjoy your rest." And Corpse Pose is just that – an opportunity after all the physical and mental work of the practice is done to rest, relax and surrender to the mat. I'll often ask my students to become aware in Savasana of the feeling of gravity gently tugging at their back body and to give in to that force, letting go of resistance. Sometimes people fall asleep in Savasana and that's just fine. It's the place where you can really let go – of the effort and physical exertion of the practice, of thinking and of judgment. Just come home and let yourself be for a few minutes. Let's give it a try.

Lie on your mat face up with your head at the top of the mat. Let your heels be about hip-width apart, but if you want you can bring them even farther apart than that. Let your toes flop toward the outside of the mat so your pinkie toes are closer to the mat than your big toes. Make sure your head is centered on your shoulders and your gaze (preferably through gently closed eyes) is straight up so

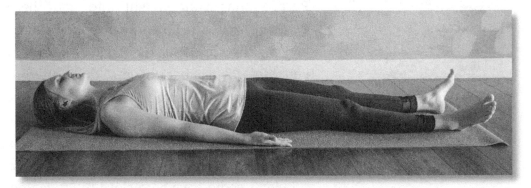

you're not lifting your chin away from your sternum, tucking it down toward the sternum or twisting your head to one side or the other. Keep your arms long and by your sides, although you can bring them out a bit if that feels right. You've got two options with the hands, either palms up (as shown in the picture) or palms down. Palms up generally feels more receptive to the gifts of Savasana. But palms down will feel more grounding. Relax the whole back body, all the way from the back of your head through the back of your shoulders and shoulder blades, the mid- and lower back, your glutes, the back of your thighs, your calves and your heels. Once you feel the straight body pose as you lie on your back, settle into your breath. Your teacher may or may not cue breathing. If they do, follow the cues. If not, either breath slowly and with intention, perhaps fixing your awareness on your navel and noticing it rise up as you breathe in and drop down as you breathe out, or let your body breathe for you and just observe the breath, watching as you breathe in and out and noticing how the process feels. Come out of Savasana slowly, gently moving your fingers and toes and then the wrists and ankles and then following the direction of your teacher to complete the yoga practice.

Plank Pose *(Kumbhakasana)*

Plank Pose (Kumbhakasana) is our classic straight body shape, oriented face-down. You probably recognize it as the top of a pushup. Both arms are reaching straight out from the shoulders and the elbows are straight. The back is flat, just like in Mountain Pose, not rounded or arched, and the hips are in a straight line with the heels and the shoulders. The head is centered between the shoulders and the neck is a natural extension of the spine, not twisted to one side or the other or arched or rounded. It helps a lot to spread your fingers wide so you can feel a little bit of a stretch in the skin on the palms. This creates a nice wide stable platform for the pose and gets you used to holding your hands that way, which you'll find useful as you learn more advanced poses, including arm balancing poses. One final tip: pressing back on the heels and reaching the top of the head, the crown, forward will help you emphasize the straight body shape of the pose and bring awareness to the length you're creating from head to toe.

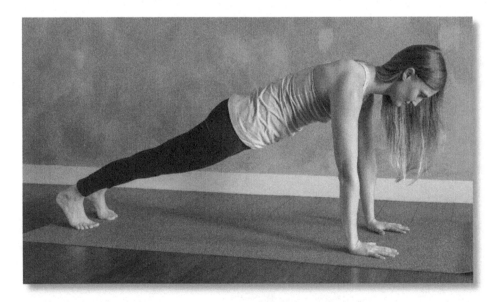

Let's give it a try. Start on your hands and knees, checking to see that your hands are under or just forward of your shoulders and your knees are right under your hips. Your hands will be about shoulder width apart and your knees will be about hip-width apart. Flatten your back and practice reaching your head forward, lengthening your neck, keeping your gaze down between your hands and pressing your tailbone back. Remembering to spread your fingers wide, press your palms, fingertips and thumbs into the mat, straightening your arms and pressing the mat away from you. Take a couple of breaths as you feel the length in your body and the strength of your arms supporting your upper body. Now pick the right knee up off the mat, straighten your right leg and step your right foot back, tucking your toes and bringing them down to the mat. Press back on the right heel and feel the straightness of the body on the right side. Finally, pick your left knee up and step your left foot back, tucking the toes and bringing them down to the mat. Make sure your feet feel even with one another and that one isn't more forward than the other. Now check that your hips are level and your whole body is straight and feel the energy moving in opposite directions: the crown of the head reaching forward, the heels pressing back and the hands pressing into the mat beneath you. Take a couple of breaths and then release your knees down to the mat to come out of the pose.

Variations: Supported Plank Pose. If it's too challenging for you to hold Plank Pose, you can perform the Pose with your knees on the mat instead of your feet.

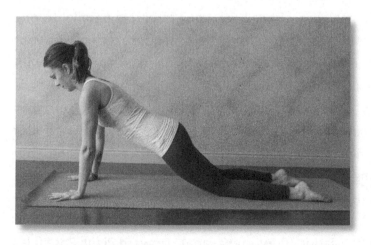

In this variation, make sure your body is straight from the crown of the head to the knees and that you aren't hinging at the hips or rounding your back. You can experiment with this variation by bending your knees once you're in the pose and lifting your feet off the mat so you're resting just on hands and knees (not pictured).

Dolphin Plank Pose variation. Dolphin Plank Pose (Makara Adho Mukha Svanasana). Dolphin Plank Pose is similar to Plank Pose. The difference is that in Dolphin Plank the forearms and elbows support the upper body instead of the hands, as is the case in Plank Pose. To come into the pose, begin on hands and knees as explained in the description of Plank Pose. Now bend both arms and bring your elbows to the mat just below your shoulders. Take a moment to flatten your back, lifting your navel toward your spine to take the arch out of your low back.

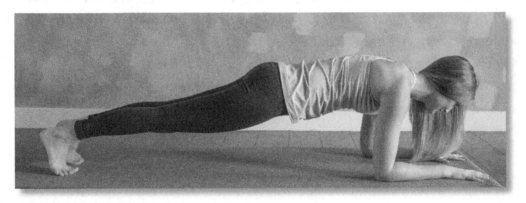

Press your forearms into the mat and either keep your forearms parallel to one another and press your palms into the mat, or bring your hands together with your palms facing one another and interlace your fingers, forming an "A" shape with your forearms. Now step your right foot back as described above for Plank Pose and then the left foot. Press back on your heels and reach the crown of your head forward, making sure your chin isn't lifted away from or pressed down toward your sternum. Make sure your hips are in a straight line with your heels and your shoulders. Take a few breaths, feel the straight body shape and when you're ready, release your knees down to the mat, coming out of the Pose.

Upward or Reverse Plank variation (Purvottanasana). Upward Plank Pose (also called Reverse Plank) is another straight body pose oriented in the supine position like Corpse Pose (Savasana). In Upward Plank, the arms reach straight behind you.

This pose is deeply challenging to the core and it's easy to find your body moving into a forward or backward curving shape instead of the straight body shape. Start seated on your mat with your legs straight and parallel to one another. Sit up nice and tall, elongating your spine and keeping your head and neck straight and your chin level. Press your palms into the mat on either side of your hips with your

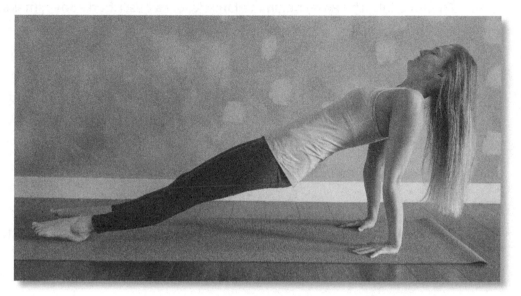

fingers facing your feet and your thumbs pointing toward one another. Slide your hands back about a foot and bring your shoulder blades together on your back. Engage your core, particularly the abs and low back, and begin to lift your hips until they're in a straight line with your shoulders and your heels. Press your heels into the mat and reach the top of your head (the crown, not the forehead) away from your heels, finding as much length as you can. Breathe deeply, imagining that you can lift the breath from your heels all the way to the top of your head on an inhale and send it back down on the exhale. Become aware of your back and correct your position if you begin to lift your hips (creating an arch in the back) or let your hips drop down (rounding your back). Note: if your wrists feel too strained in this pose with your fingers pointing toward the toes, perform the pose with your fingers pointing out and the thumbs pointing toward your feet.

Side Plank Pose *(Vasisthasana)*

Side Plank Pose (Vasisthasana) is the straight body shape with the body oriented on the side and the arms reaching straight out to the side from the shoulders. To move into the Pose, begin in Plank Pose, as described above, making

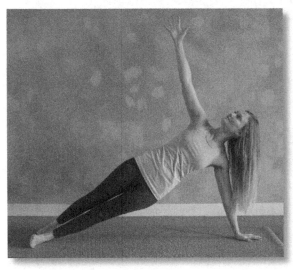

sure your hands are a few inches in front of your shoulders instead of directly under them. Check in to make sure your body is aligned in the straight shape in Plank Pose with your feet about hip-width apart. Now roll over onto the outside (pinkie toe) edge of your left foot and the inside (big toe) edge of your right foot, making sure the front of the left foot is at least an inch behind the heel of your right foot. Keeping your body straight and trying to avoid twisting your torso, transfer your weight to your left hand, spreading the fingers wide on the mat, and reach your right arm up and out from the shoulder so it's about 180 degrees from your

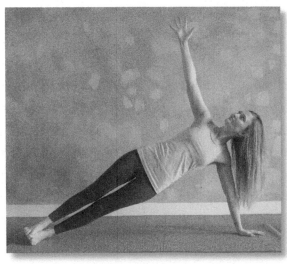

left arm, which is now supporting the weight of your upper body. Keep your head reaching away from your feet and lengthening the whole body. Once in the pose, bring your awareness to your hips and notice if your hips are lifted up beyond the straight body shape (which would create a side curve to the right) or if the hips are drooping down (which would create a side curve to the left) and correct the shape as needed. If you feel solid in that version of Side Plank, try the Pose stacking your right foot on top of your left, as shown in the last picture on the previous page, so that only the outside edge (the pinkie toe side) of your left foot is touching the mat. When you're done, rotate back to Plank Pose and then move to Side Plank Pose on the other side. Note: when I teach this Pose I make sure the student's hand is a few inches forward of the shoulder so the arm and torso form a 90-degree angle. If the hand is directly below the shoulder on the mat, the angle between the arm and the torso will be less than 90 degrees and that can be hard on the shoulder muscles.

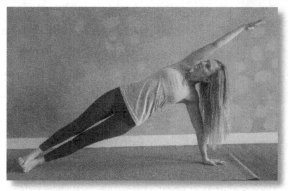

If you want more out of the Pose and to more deeply challenge your core, try reaching the upper arm forward with your palm down instead of reaching it up toward the sky.

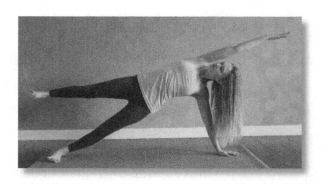

Even more challenge can be added by lifting your upper leg at the same time as your arm and reaching the upper leg toward the back of the room as you stretch the fingertips of your raised hand forward in opposition to the raised leg.

Variations:

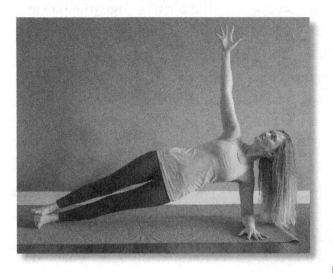

Side Plank on the Elbow. Just as we can perform a Plank Pose on the elbows instead of the hands, we can do the same thing with Side Plank Pose. Start in Plank on the elbows, as explained under Plank Pose, above. Now walk your elbows forward about an inch so the elbows are in front of the shoulders instead of right below them. Keeping the elbow bent at 90 degrees, pivot on the left elbow and bring your left forearm so that it's parallel to the front of the mat. Let the whole forearm and the palm of the left hand bear the weight of your upper body as you roll over onto the outside edge of the left foot, as described above for Side Plank Pose, and then proceed with the Pose as you would in Side Plank.

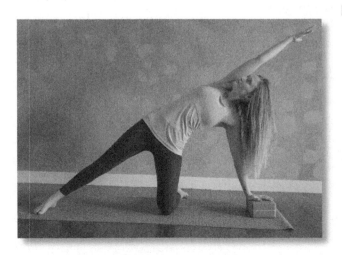

Supported Side Plank Pose. This variation is much more forgiving to the core because your hips are supported by the knee of the bottom leg. Start on hands and knees. Walk your hands forward a couple of inches. Step the right foot back, straighten the right leg and bring the inside edge (big toe side) of the right foot to the mat. At this point your left hip should be right over your left knee, which should still be on the mat. Pivoting on the left knee, keep your left leg bent at 90-degrees and swing your left foot around to your left until the shin of that leg is parallel to the front edge of the mat. Now open the hips to the right, stacking your right hip over your left, pressing into the left knee as you do that. At the same time, ground into your left hand, spreading your fingers wide and reach your right hand either up to the sky or bring it by the right ear as shown in the picture.

Supine Pigeon Pose *(Supta Kapotasana).* Supine Pigeon Pose

(sometimes called Dead Pigeon or Eye of the Needle) opens the hip joint. It can be challenging to get into, particularly if your hips are tight. When not done properly, it may seem like a curved body shape with your torso curving forward. But when done properly, you'll see that it is clearly based on the straight body shape, with the knees bent and one leg externally rotated to open the hip on that side.

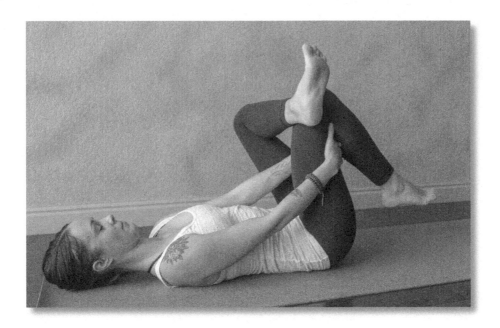

Begin on your back in Corpse Pose, noticing the straight body shape. Keep a flat back as you bend both of your knees and bring them up toward your chest while lifting both feet off the mat, making sure to press your tailbone down toward the mat. Bring the left ankle to the top of the right knee so the center of your foot lines up with the kneecap. With your left hand reach into the figure A formed by your legs and with the right hand reach behind your right thigh, eventually bringing your hands together behind your right leg just above the knee and interlacing your fingers. Now gently pull your right knee toward you as you press your left knee away. Check your hips to make sure both are pressing into the mat and that your hips are square to the short edge of the mat. Now check again to make sure your back is flat and straight. If you've rounded your back, either by lifting your hips off the mat or by lifting your shoulders, allow them to release down to the mat and come back to the straight body shape. Also check your head and neck, making sure your neck is extending straight back from your spine and your head isn't lifted up off the mat or turned to one side or the other. Finally, check your chin to make sure it's level and not reaching toward your sternum or lifting up and away from the sternum. Take a few breaths in the Pose and then release your hands and feet and then practice the Pose on the other side.

Child's Pose *(Balasana)*

You will find yourself in Child's Pose in most classes and it's also a wonderful resting pose to retreat to if you find yourself fatigued during a yoga practice. There are two variations of the Pose, one with knees together and one with knees wide and the torso draped between the thighs. The wide-kneed variation is a straight body shape and the Pose done with the knees together, which we'll learn later, is a curved body shape with the torso bending forward. For now let's focus on the version of Child's Pose with the knees apart and a flat back.

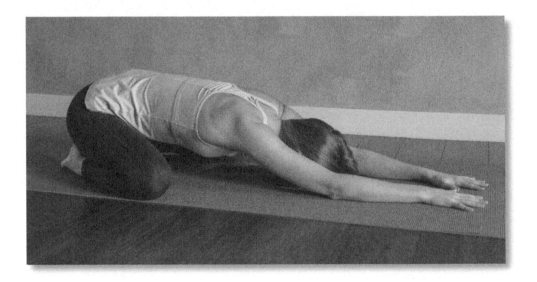

To begin, kneel on the mat with knees together, hips on the heels, big toes touching and your hands palms-down on your thighs. As you inhale feel your spine lengthen toward the sky as the top of your head rises and your neck lengthens. Keep your gaze forward and your chin level. Keeping the long spine, bring your hands to the mat and keeping the big toes touching, bring your knees apart as much as is comfortable, perhaps to the edges of the mat, and then hinge at your hips as you let your torso come down toward the mat draping between your thighs. Reach your arms out in front of you, stretching out from your shoulders. Pause for a moment and feel the straight shape from your tailbone to your fingertips, making sure your neck is extending straight and is not arched, rounded or twisted. If you feel any arching or rounding in your back, take a moment to try to straighten the back.

If your torso won't come all the way down to the mat between your thighs or you don't feel you can find the straight shape and that the back or neck is curved, either rounded forward or arched back, let's do the Pose with a prop. Use either a long bolster (or thick pillow) or one or two folded blankets and place them under your torso, running from your navel to just below your chin. Let your belly and chest rest on the prop and make sure you can feel the straight body shape. Note that depending on the thickness of your prop, you may need to rest your forehead on a prop of a different thickness to maintain the straight shape all the way from your tailbone through the crown of your head. Once you've found the straight shape in the Pose, enjoy a few rounds of breath. When you want to come out of the Pose, rise back up to kneeling, bring your knees back together and let your palms rest on your thighs.

Easy Pose *(Sukhasana)*

Yoga classes often begin in a seated position and so let's learn a basic seated posture, Easy Pose. To begin, come to a seat on your mat and cross your legs so your knees are wide and one heel is tucked in close to your pubic bone and the opposite foot is under that knee. Press your sitting bones into the mat and as you breathe in, allow your spine to lengthen and the crown of your head to rise up

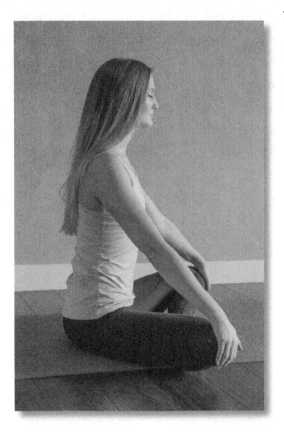

toward the sky. Keep your chin level and your gaze forward. Make sure your back is flat and not rounded or arched. Remember this is a straight body pose (with the legs bent at the hip and externally rotated). If your hips are tight and your knees sit quite a bit above the mat, sit on a prop. Either a folded blanket, a block or a bolster will do. Depending on how tight your hips are, you may need to elevate your hips up to six or nine inches. The effect of elevating your hips will be to increase the angle between your thighs and your upper body. Without the prop, that angle is about 90 degrees. With the prop, the angle might be up to 120 degrees. If you're using the prop, pay special attention to your back, making sure it's straight and long.

Variation. A common variation you'll encounter is to perform Easy Pose with a spinal twist. For this variation, come into the pose as described above and let your awareness rest for a moment on the straight shape of the spine. Keep that shape as you twist to the left, bringing your left shoulder so it's pointing more or

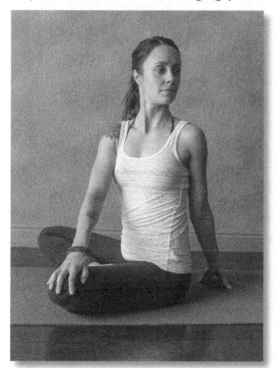

less toward the back of the room. Allow your gaze to follow the twist so you'll end up looking over your left shoulder. With each inhale, find a little bit more length in your spine, keeping the chin level. On an exhale come out of the twist and back to center. Breathe in and then twist to the other side on an exhale. Keep your attention fixed on lengthening the spine.

Runner's Lunge Pose *(Ardha Hanumanasana)*

You will probably do Runner's Lunge Pose in most yoga classes you take. The basic shape is similar to the stance a sprinter takes on the starting blocks. Let's practice two different ways of getting into the Pose. Stand at the front of your mat with your feet parallel to one another and about hip-width apart. Reach both arms overhead into Extended Mountain Pose and then, hinging at the hips, bring both hands to the mat just in front of your feet. Bend your left knee as you step your right foot back far enough that your left knee is bent to about 90 degrees. Stay up on the ball of your right foot with your toes tucked and make sure your right leg is straight. Press back on your right heel and reach the crown of your head forward toward the front of the room. Notice that your right heel, your hips, your shoulders

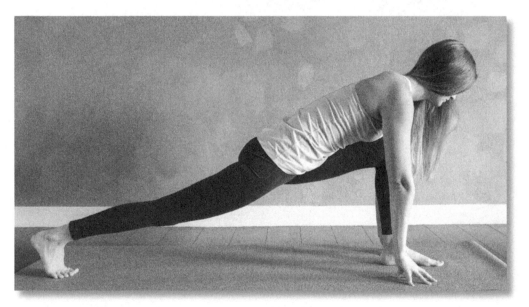

and your head are all in a straight line, the classic straight body shape. The only difference between Runner's Lunge Pose and Plank Pose is that the left leg and knee are bent so the sole of the left foot is resting on the mat and supporting some of your weight. You can confirm this by engaging your core, emphasizing the straight body shape, and stepping your right foot back so it meets the left. Notice now that you're in Plank Pose and the only change you've made is that you've straightened your right leg. Come out of Runner's Lunge Pose (ignoring the step back into Plank Pose) by stepping your right foot forward to meet your left and rising back up to Mountain Pose, keeping your back flat and hinging at your hips. Now practice the same thing on the other side, stepping the left foot back this time.

Another common way to enter Runner's Lunge Pose is from Downward Facing Dog Pose, which you'll learn in the next section on Hinged Body Poses. After you learn Downward Facing Dog, come into that pose, noticing the hinged body shape hinged at the hips. Lift your left leg slightly as you glide forward so your shoulders are directly over or even a little bit in front of your hands. Then step your left foot forward between your hands and bring your hips down so they're in a straight line with your shoulders and your right heel. Ground into your left foot, press both hands into the mat, reach the top of your head forward and press back on your right heel with your toes tucked, making sure that your right leg is straight. Now notice that you've found the straight body shape, with the variation that the left leg is bent at the hip and the knee. After enjoying a few breaths and feeling the straightness of your body in the Pose, lift your hips a bit and step your left foot back to Plank Pose and then lift your hips back to Downward Facing Dog Pose. Take a little break if you need to and then do the Pose on the other side, stepping the right foot forward this time.

Warrior II *(Virabhadrasana II)*

Warrior II, our next straight body pose, is named after the fierce warrior Virabhadra. If you look carefully at the picture below, you'll notice the characteristics of the straight body shape. The shoulders are directly over the hips, the back is flat and the head is centered on the shoulders. However, the Pose makes a number of modifications to our simple straight body shape. The left leg,

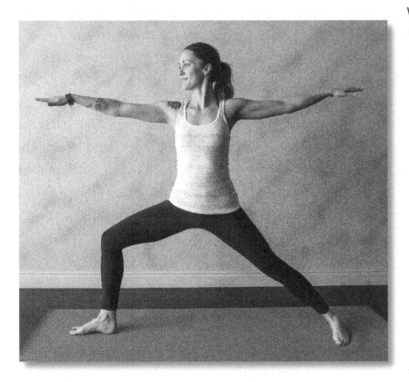

while remaining straight, is angled toward the back of the mat and rotates in the hip joint. The right leg is rotated even more deeply in the hip joint and the right knee is bent to about 90 degrees. Both arms are reaching out from the shoulder joints and the neck is twisted 90-degrees so the gaze is forward over the extended right hand. In spite of those modifications, can you still see the straight body shape?

Let's move into the Warrior II by starting in Runner's Lunge Pose with your right foot forward and your left foot back. Spin the heel of the left foot down to the mat so the toes point to the left side of the mat. You should be in a wide stance with your right knee bent up to 90 degrees and the feet 3 to 4 feet apart. However, if that doesn't feel sustainable, shorten your stance a little bit, reducing the bend in the right knee. Roll your left foot toward the back of the mat so you feel grounded into the outside edge of that foot, the pinkie toe side. Now raise your arms and stretch your hands apart from one another with palms facing down, feeling a little stretch between your collar bones. Make sure your arms are reaching in opposition to one another. Finally, keep your chin level, but rotate your head so your gaze is forward over your outstretched right hand. Check your alignment and notice that you have retained the essentials of the straight body shape, with your shoulders over your hips and your head centered over your pubic bone. Make sure you're not leaning forward or creating an arch in or rounding your back.

As you breathe in, draw the breath up from your pubic bone to the crown of your head and feel the length of your upper body. As you exhale, send the breath back down to the pubic bone. Circulate the breath this way a few times. When you're ready to come out of the Pose, bring your hands down on either side of your right foot and come up onto the ball of your left foot, returning to Runner's Lunge Pose. Then step your left foot forward and rise into Mountain Pose. When you're ready, move into Runner's Lunge Pose with the right foot back and proceed with Warrior II on the other side.

Warrior III *(Virabhadrasana III)*

Warrior III is a challenging balancing pose done on one leg. Can you see the straight body shape in the picture of the Pose below? It looks just like Extended Mountain Pose but with the body parallel to the mat and standing on one leg. Notice that with the exception of the leg you're standing on, the hips are in line with the feet, the shoulders in line with the hips, the head right in the center and the arms reaching directly overhead.

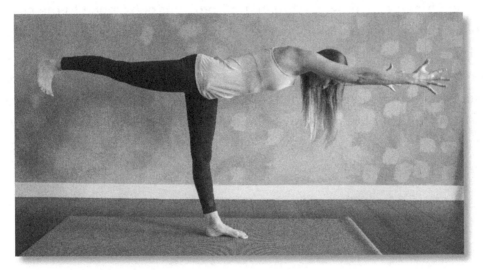

Let's practice Warrior III. Begin in Mountain Pose and then reach your arms up and overhead into Extended Mountain Pose. Transfer your weight to your left foot and begin to allow a little bend in the left knee. Concentrate on hinging at your left hip as you lengthen by reaching your hands and your right foot away from one another. Maintain the straight body shape as you eventually bring your entire straight body parallel to the floor and then straighten your left knee. Keep reaching the crown of your head out from your shoulders and avoid tucking your chin or lifting it away from your sternum. The more you lengthen through the whole body the more stable the pose will feel and the less likely you'll be to either round your back (dropping your head and foot down toward the mat) or arch (lifting your head, hands or foot away from the mat). After a few breaths, bring your right foot to the mat and, hinging at the hip, return to Extended Mountain Pose. Then release your hands and bring them down to your sides in Mountain Pose. When you're ready, move into the Pose on the other side.

Variations. Warrior III is sometimes done with different arm positions. Having the arms outstretched, as described above, is the most challenging version of the pose and engages the core most deeply. Other variations may be less energetic. Bringing your hands to your heart and pressing your palms together is an option. In this variation recognize the tendency to arch the back and lift the

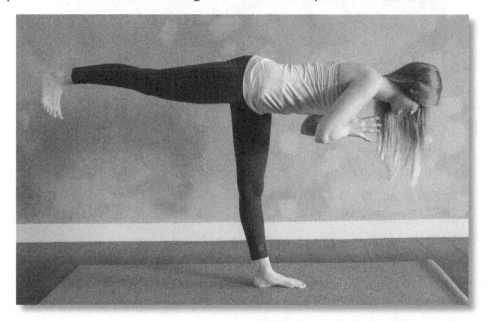

chin; counter that by keeping your chin neutral and continually reaching out through the crown of your head. Balance usually seems easier in this variation because the hands pressing together, drawing energy to the mid-line of the body which produces a centering and grounding effect.

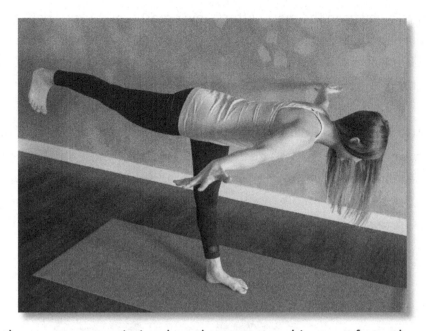

Another common variation has the arms reaching out from the shoulders mimicking the wings of an airplane. Begin with the arms that way and then hinge at the hip into the Pose. Keep reaching your hands apart from one another with the palms facing down, creating as much wingspan as you can. The airplane version of Warrior III is probably the most accessible if balance is a challenge. Just notice that you are reaching in four directions at once, north with the crown of the head, south with the lifted foot and east and west with the hands.

A final variation you will want to try if you're struggling with balance is a 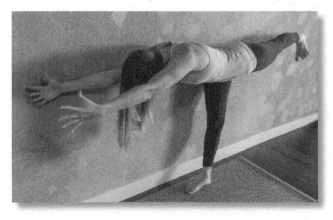 supported Warrior III. For this variation, arrange your mat so the long side is against a wall. Stand on the mat in Mountain Pose with your right foot a couple inches from the wall and the rest of the right side of your body gently touching the wall. Reach your arms up and overhead into Extended Mountain Pose. Transfer your weight to your right foot and move into the Pose as described above, but letting your right hip, shoulder and arm rest gently against the wall. With the wall providing support you can let go of concerns about balance and feel the straight body shape in the Pose, with your fingertips reaching forward and your left foot stretching back. After a few breaths release to Extended Mountain Pose and then to bring your hands back down by your side. Then turn around the other way and try the Pose on the other side.

Tree Pose *(Vrksasana)*

Tree Pose is another upright straight body shaped balancing pose. By now you recognize the straight body shape and you can see that Tree Pose is basically Mountain Pose with one leg externally rotated, lifted at the hip and bent at the knee. In addition, the arms aren't by the sides as in Mountain Pose, but the elbows are bent and the palms are brought together at the heart.

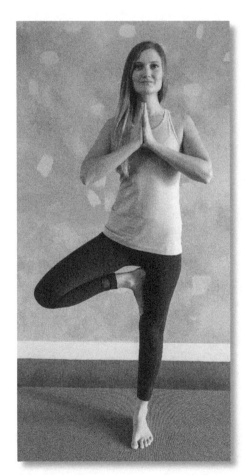

To move into Tree Pose, begin in Mountain Pose with your arms lose and by your sides. Transfer your weight to your left foot, making sure the weight is distributed evenly between your toes, the ball of your foot and both sides of your heel. Pick your right foot up and bring the sole of the foot to the inside of your left leg, anywhere from the ankle to groin, but avoiding the knee. Feel free to lift your foot into position with your hand if you need to. Bring your hands to your heart and press your palms lightly together. Press the sole of your right foot into the inside of your leg and at the same time press your leg into the sole of your foot. This creates dynamic tension and will provide stability in the Pose. Reach the crown of your head up toward the sky and keep your chin level. Try to avoid twisting your torso and keep your hips right over your feet and your shoulders over your hips. Depending on the flexibility in your hips, see if you can press the right knee off to the right so that its directly in line with both hips. Take a few more breaths in the Pose and then release back to Mountain Pose. When you're ready, practice the Pose standing on the right foot.

Variations.

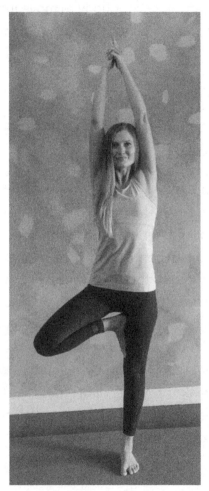

Sometimes Tree pose is done with the arms stretched overhead. Begin as suggested above and once you feel stable in the Pose, reach your arms straight up and overhead. Your hands can be apart with the palms facing one another or you can bring your hands together and interlace your fingers, pointing your index fingers straight up to the sky.

If you feel stable in Tree Pose, release the hands and try swaying your arms side to side overhead, like the branches of a tree blowing gently in the wind.

If you're having trouble balancing in Tree Pose, there are two different levels of support you can try. First, try the Pose against the wall. Stand with your back to the wall, heels a couple inches away from the wall and your glutes and shoulder blades resting gently against the wall. Now pick up your right foot and bring it to the inside of your left leg, as described above, and bring your hands to your heart, lightly pressing your palms together. The wall will support you in the Pose and you can concentrate on lengthening up through the spine and through the crown of the head. Once you feel grounded, see if you can allow your body to move just a bit off the wall and stay grounded in the standing foot. Practice this way until the balance comes to you.

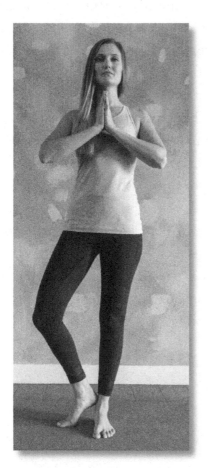

If you don't have a wall handy, here's another option: standing on your left foot, externally rotate your right leg so the toes on your right foot point 90-degrees to your right. Then bring the back of the heel of your right foot to the inside of the ankle of your left foot and let the big toe of your right foot rest on the mat. Concentrate on pressing your right foot into the mat and lengthening through your whole body. Think of your right foot as a sort of kickstand, just giving your balance a little extra support.

Triangle Pose *(Trikonasana)*

A few common yoga poses don't fit neatly into one category or another. Triangle Pose is one of those. But I think it's best thought of as a straight body shape, mainly because the essence of the Pose is lengthening the spine from the tailbone through the torso from the upper hip to the crown of the head. If you look at the picture of the Pose below you can see at least two triangles, one formed by the mat and the two legs and the other formed by the forward leg, the torso and the arm reaching down to the mat. Triangle Pose is similar to Warrior II, which is a straight body shape, but with the upper body parallel to the mat instead of upright and the right knee bent instead of straight.

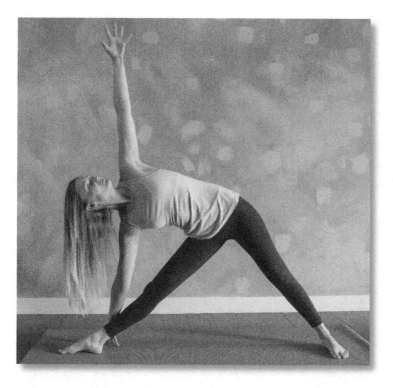

Begin in Mountain Pose near the back of your mat and facing the long edge of the mat. Step your right foot toward the front of the mat 3 or 4 feet and pivot on the heel of the right foot so your toes point to the front of the mat. Keep both legs straight and lengthen through the spine as you reach your arms out to a "T," raising them so they end up parallel to the mat. Reach the right arm forward as far as you can, keeping your spine long and straight and hinging at the right hip until your torso is at an angle anywhere between 45 degrees and level with the mat. Allow your right arm to drop straight down as you reach your left arm up to the sky. Ground into your left foot as you bring the left side of your hip over the right as much as possible without strain. If it feels better, let the left hip drop and to the left, which will introduce a little bit of a spinal twist. Continue lengthening your spine and reaching out through the crown of your head. You can keep your gaze out or turn your head, twisting your neck so your gaze is up to the sky. Come out of the Pose as you entered it and step the right foot back to Mountain Pose. Then practice Triangle Pose on the other side.

Section 2 - Hinged Body Poses

Downward Facing Dog Pose *(Adho Mukha Svanasana)*

Of all the yoga poses based on the hinged body shape, Downward Facing Dog is certainly the most well-known. It will be the very rare yoga practice that doesn't' include this Pose. Notice from the picture that the shape of Downward Facing Dog is unmistakably the hinged body shape with the upper and lower parts of the body hinged at 90 degrees. The arms are outstretched, forming a long straight line from the hips to the hands, without any rounding or arching of the back. Depending on the flexibility in your ankles and hamstrings, which will become more mobile with more practice, the heels may or may not reach all the way to the mat. Also, if the hamstrings are tight you may not be able to straighten the legs. That's just fine. A little bend in the knees is perfectly ok as long as you keep your back flat and avoid rounding. Finally, notice that the chin is in the neutral position, not lifting away from the sternum or pressing down toward the sternum.

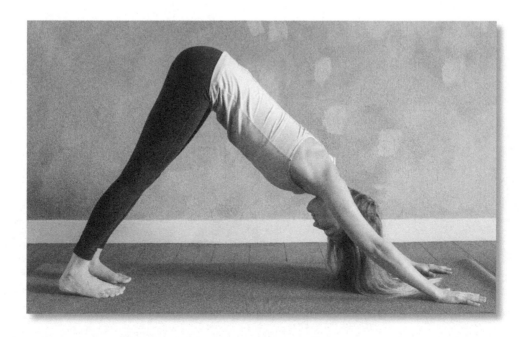

Begin on hands and knees. Flatten your back by reaching the top of your head forward (without lifting your chin), lengthen the spine by reaching your tailbone back and bring your navel to your spine to take any excessive arch out of the lumbar portion of your spine. Walk your hands forward about six inches and then tuck your toes and lift your hips, straightening your legs. On an in-breath, spread your fingers wide, press your hands into the mat like you're trying to stretch the front of the mat forward and press your tailbone up and back while you continue to hug your navel toward your spine. Hold the pose for a few breaths, continuing to lengthen from the hands pressing into the mat to the tailbone and from the hips to the heels. When you're ready to come out of the Pose, bend both knees and bring them to the mat, returning to hands and knees.

Dolphin Pose *(Makarasana or Ardha Pincha Mayurasana)*

Dolphin Pose is similar to Downward Facing Dog. The main difference is that in Dolphin Pose the forearms are resting on the mat instead of the hands. But there are some other subtleties that we'll explore.

Begin on hands and knees. Just as you did preparing for Downward Facing Dog, flatten your back by reaching the top of your head forward (without lifting your chin), lengthen your spine by reaching your tailbone back and bring your navel to your spine to take the arch out of your lower back. Bring your elbows to the mat right under your shoulders. It's important not to separate your elbows more than shoulder width. To check on that distance, pivot on both forearms and grasp the left elbow with the right hand and the right elbow with the left hand. If you can't easily reach the opposite elbow with your hand, then your elbows are too far apart

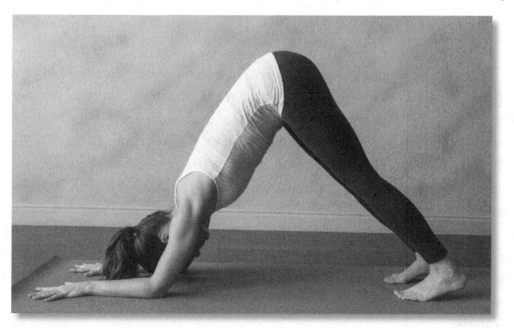

and you need to bring them closer together. Once you've gotten the elbows properly spaced bring the forearms back to the mat. You can do one of two things with your forearms: either keep them parallel to one another with the palms pressing into the mat and the fingers spread wide or bring your hands together forming an "A" with your forearms and interlacing your fingers or making a fist with one hand and grasping the fist with the other hand. Try both options and see which one feels most natural and comfortable to you.

Now press your elbows, forearms and hands into the mat. Then tuck your toes, straighten your legs and begin to walk both feet forward until your upper and lower body form approximately a 90-degree angle. Straighten your knees as much as you can (without hyperextending), but if your hamstrings are tight, bent knees are fine too. Reach your tailbone up and back, extending your spine and check to see that your shoulders are behind your elbows so that your upper arms are in a straight line with your torso. Relax your head, but avoid lifting or tucking your chin. Keep it neutral. Enjoy a few breaths in Dolphin Pose, becoming aware that your upper and lower body is hinged at the hips and forming about a 90-degree angle. When you're ready to come out of the Pose, bring your knees back down to the mat and press your hips back to your heels into Child's Pose.

A couple more things to be mindful of in Dolphin Pose. It's common to want to lift your head up in the Pose and gaze forward. If you do that, you are likely to bring an arch into your spine. Better to leave your chin neutral, lengthening your neck and reaching out through the top of your head and the tailbone. If your forehead is touching the mat, it's probably because your elbows have moved too far apart which lets the head droop down toward the mat. If so, come out of the Pose and bring the elbows closer together and try again. Dolphin Pose is a big hamstring stretch for some people. If your hamstrings are too tight to straighten your legs, you can bend your knees a little, making sure you keep the length in your spine and avoid rounding your back. Don't force yourself into the pose with tight hamstrings because that will cause the low back to round and you'll lose the hinged body shape.

Standing Half Lift Pose *(Ardha Uttanasana)*

Standing Half Lift Pose is often done as part of a sequence, usually sandwiched between two Forward Fold Poses, which we'll learn in the Curved Body Pose Section later in this book. Notice the Standing Half Lift Pose is our classic hinged body shape, just like Downward Facing Dog, only done standing with the upper body parallel to the mat. A little bit of balance comes into play in this Pose and we'll pay close attention to how the weight is distributed between the front and back of the feet.

Let's begin in Mountain Pose, facing the front of your mat with your feet parallel to one another and a little bit less than hip-width apart. Bring your

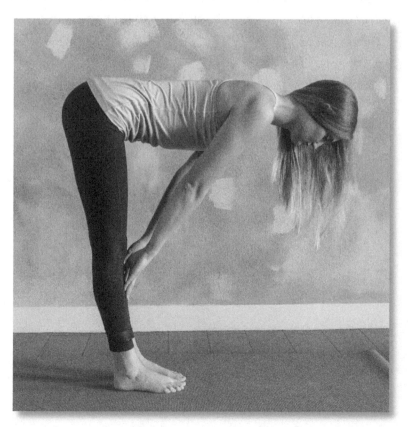

attention to your feet and press down on the toe mounds as well as the inside and outside part of both heels. Notice that your weight is distributed evenly on both feet and front to back on each foot, as well as the inside and outside edges of both feet. Inhale deeply and let your spine elongate, but without lifting the chin, reaching the crown of your head toward the sky. Engage your core, particularly the abs and your low back. Hinging at the hips and keeping your back flat and legs straight, begin to slowly bring your torso down until it's parallel with the mat and your upper body forms a 90-degree angle with your legs. At the same time, bring your palms to the top of your shins, right below the knees, and press your palms into the shins and straighten your arms. If you press your palms even more deeply into your shins you'll find that you're pressing your hips and tailbone back and this will help lengthen your back. Reach your shoulders apart from one another and try to flatten your back between the shoulder blades, avoiding rounding the shoulders. Bring your weight forward into the balls of your feet and the toes, taking most of the weight off your heels. Take a few moments to feel into the hinged body shape, taking care that your back is flat and not rounded or arched. If you feel arching, lift your navel toward your spine. If you feel rounding lift your chin a little away from your chest and reach your forehead forward to remove the rounding. Then keep that shape and bring your chin back to the neutral position.

Staff Pose *(Dandasana)*

You will recognize Staff Pose as our hinged body shape in a seated orientation. Staff Pose is commonly done before moving into various different seated forward folds as well as before Upward or Reverse Plank Pose, which you practiced in the straight body pose section. Come to a seat on the mat with your legs straight and parallel to one another. Press your heels away from you and make sure your toes are pointing straight up. Press down on your sitting bones and then press your hands into the mat just outside of each hip. Notice how pressing your hands into the mat allows your spine to lengthen and your heart to rise. Reach the crown of

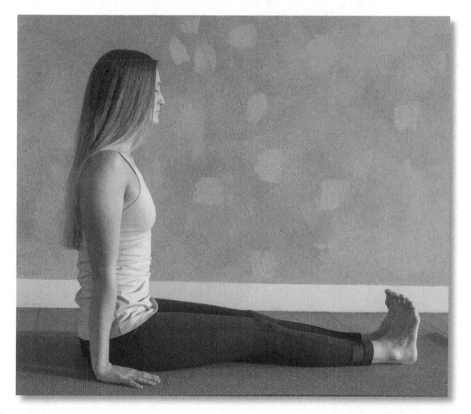

your head toward the sky, let your shoulders soften down and reach your ears away from your shoulders. Close your eyes and allow yourself to feel the hinged body shape, feeling the extension from the sitting bones up through the crown of the head and from the hips forward through your heels.

Variation. Extended Staff Pose (Utthita Dandasana). Perform Staff Pose as described above and then reach your arms up and overhead, palms facing one another and stretching your fingers toward the sky. It's common for an arch to creep into the back in this Pose. Resist the urge and maintain a flat back by bringing your navel to your spine and dropping the low ribs down toward your pelvic bone.

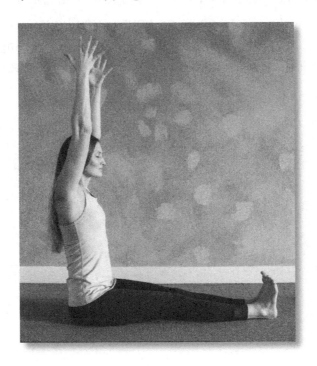

Legs up the Wall Pose *(Viparita Karani)*

Legs up the Wall Pose is a very calming posture. I love doing it for five minutes or so at the beginning of my yoga practice, particularly the supported variation described below. It's a mild, easily maintained inversion that calms the body and the mind. Notice that this is a classic hinged body shape in the supine (face up) orientation. Lie down on your back on your mat, with your legs straight, parallel

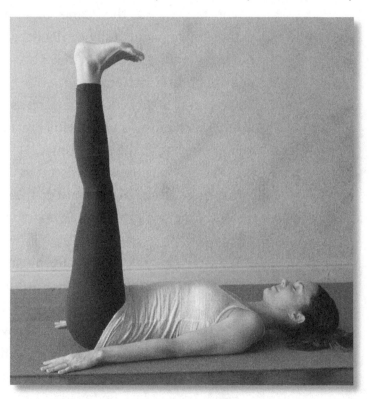

and your feet about hip-width apart. With your arms straight and by your side, rotate your palms so they face down. If you can, keep your legs straight and lift your legs so your heels end up directly above your hips. If that's too difficult, bend the knees first. Press your heels toward the sky as you press your sacrum gently into the mat, lengthening through your lower body. Also flatten your back, pressing the back of the shoulders, the shoulder blades and the mid and lower back lightly into the mat. Enjoy three to five breaths as you embody the hinged body shape, extending your feet toward the sky and the crown of your head toward the front of the mat.

Variations. Supported Legs up the Wall Pose. There are two ways to do the supported variation of this Pose, against the wall or with a strap. For the wall variation, bring the short edge of your mat to the wall, lay down on the mat on your side, hug your knees into your chest with your butt pressing gently against the wall.

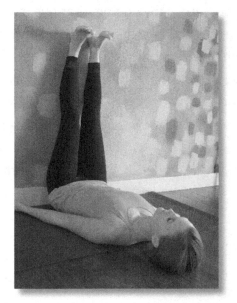

Then roll over onto your back, straighten your legs and let your heels rest against the wall, keeping your legs parallel. As above, press your sacrum into the mat and press your heels up, lengthening the lower body. At the same time, feel extension in your spine, lengthening between your glutes and the crown of your head and flattening out your back. You can stay in this position as long as you like. Five minutes is wonderfully relaxing and energizing at the same time.

The second support option is to use a cotton yoga strap. You'll want to find the longest strap you can and if what you have isn't long enough, you can couple two

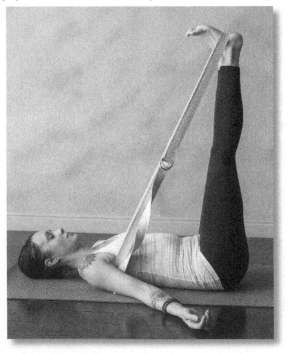

straps together. (Note: I've also used nylon ribbon tie-down straps in a pinch). Sitting on the mat, make a big loop with the strap and position the strap on your back, just under your armpits. With your feet together, bring the strap to the insteps of both of your feet, straighten your legs and flatten your back into Staff Pose. Now tighten (or loosen) the strap until it's taught. Then bend your knees as you drop your back down to the mat, keeping tension on the strap so it stays in place. With the strap in place, flatten your back and straighten your legs so your feet are held more or less directly over your hips by the strap. Remain in the supported Pose as long as you like, trying to feel the Pose and not worrying too much about the strap. When you're ready to come out of the Pose, bend your knees and you can then remove the strap and set it aside.

Boat Pose *(Navasana)*

Another obvious example of the hinged body shape, Boat Pose strengthens the core muscles (the abs, lower back and glutes) and the quadriceps. It also requires considerable balance, focus and concentration. It's easy to allow the back to round in the Pose. So continually remind yourself that the back remains straight and flat.

Begin in Staff Pose and then bend both knees, bringing the soles of the feet to the mat and slide your feet toward your body until your heels are about 14 inches from your glutes. Keeping your back flat, begin to lean back and let your feet lift off the mat at the same time. Continue leaning back until you are balancing on the three points created by your left and right sitting bones and your tailbone. When you feel stable there, begin to lift your feet until the legs are straight. At the same time

reach the top of the head up and back, lengthening your spine. Keep your chin in a neutral position, trying not to tuck it in toward your sternum or lift it up away from your chest. Keeping your arms straight, reach forward out of the shoulders with the arms parallel to the mat. Once you've found the shape and are balanced in the Pose, take a moment or two to notice where your muscles are straining to maintain the Pose and see if you can relax the effort just a little bit, maybe just 10% or 15%, and still maintain the same shape. Come back to your breath and let the breath help you lengthen from the hips to the crown of your head and from the hips to your heels or toes. When you're ready to come out of the Pose, bend your knees and bring your feet to the mat and bring your back forward to your starting position.

Variations: Half Boat Pose (Ardha Navasana). If you're struggling to maintain the shape in Boat Pose, try Half Boat Pose instead until you build up your core

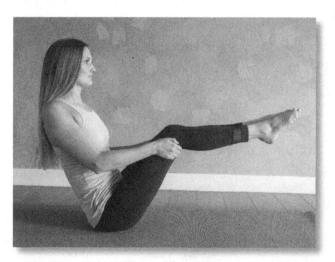

strength. Start as described above for Boat Pose, but bring your hands under your knees. With your arms bent, rock back until you're balanced on your sitting bones and tailbone and then lift your feet until your shins are parallel to the mat. Keep your back flat and your chin in a neutral position and press your knees away from your hips, creating dynamic tension with the arms. As you build core strength, try straightening your legs while still supporting them with your arms and removing your hands from your knees while keeping the knees bent in the Pose.

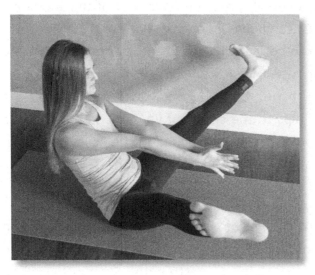

Wide-Legged Boat Pose. If you'd like to test core strength and get a little different feeling in the abs, try the wide legged variation of Boat Pose. Come into Boat Pose as described above and then bring your feet as far apart as you like, bringing your palms together and reaching your arms forward. Make sure you keep your back flat as there's a tendency for this variation to cause rounding of both the lower back (because the legs are spreading out) and the upper back (because the shoulders tend to round forward as the arms reach forward). Resist the rounding by lifting your heart and the pulling your shoulders up and back and away from your ears.

Supported Boat Pose. This is another favorite of mine. Use a yoga strap to provide support in the pose. This requires a long strap (or two shorter straps connected together). Make a big loop in the strap and apply it in the same way we learned for Legs up the Wall Pose, above. Once seated with the strap, bring your hands to the mat in front of your hips and press into the mat so your feet begin to lift as you lean back. Keep tension on the strap by maintaining a

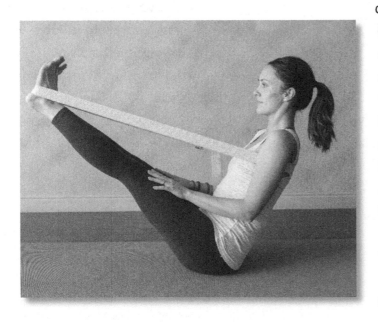

long spine and flat back and pressing the soles of your feet into the strap as you move into a balanced position. Once there, let go of all muscular control, except what you need to stay balanced. It's truly wondrous to experience Boat Pose without the core engagement and just concentrate on flattening everything out and extending from the hips both in the direction of the feet and the head. When you're ready to come out of the supported Pose, bend your knees and release the strap and come back to a seat. Note: if the strap bothers your feet or you're troubled by the feeling that your feet are being crushed together by the pressure of the strap, you can do the Pose with shoes on or place a block the long way across the insteps of both feet.

Three Legged Dog Pose *(Eka Pada Adho Mukha Svanasana)*

Three Legged Dog Pose can be seen as a variation of Downward Facing Dog. You can see in the picture below that the basic shape of the Pose is the same as Downward Facing Dog, with the exception that one leg is lifted. Other than that change, it's the very recognizable hinged body shape of Downward Facing Dog.

Begin on hands and knees. Flatten your back by reaching the top of your head forward (without lifting the chin), lengthen your spine by reaching your tailbone back and bring your navel to the spine to take any excessive arch out of the lumbar portion of your spine. Walk your hands forward about six inches and then tuck your

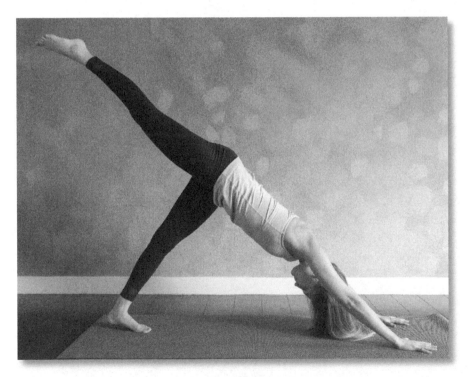

toes and lift your hips, straightening your legs. As you breathe in spread your fingers wide, press your hands into the mat like you're trying to stretch the front of the mat forward and press your tailbone up and back while you continue to hug your navel toward your spine, coming into Downward Facing Dog. On an in-breath lift your right leg up while keeping both legs straight. Stretch through the toes of the lifted foot and press down on the heel of the other leg while you continue to reach your tailbone up and back. When you're ready, exhale and bring your right foot down, returning to Downward Facing Dog. Then bend your knees and return to hands and knees. When you're ready, practice the Pose on the other side, lifting your left leg up this time.

Variation. You'll encounter a very common variation of this Pose by bending the knee and opening the hips to the side. Let's give it a try. Come into Three Legged Dog Pose as described above. Now bend your left knee and begin to open

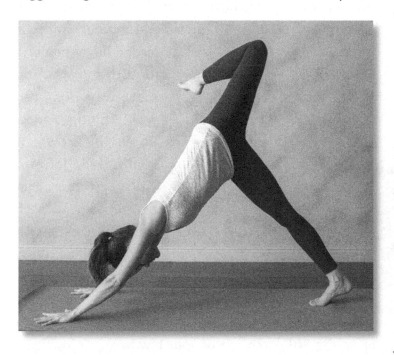

your hips to the left, stacking the left hip on top of the right hip and moving into a spinal twist. Press your left knee up and away from your hands pressing into the mat. Keep your shoulders square to the front of the mat. Otherwise you'll be negating the effect of the twisting in the torso. When you're ready to come out of the Pose, square your hips to the mat and bring your left foot back to the mat, returning to Downward Facing Dog. Then explore the variation on the right side.

Table Pose *(Bharmanasana)*

Table Pose (Bharmanasana) is a common pose often practiced in the transition to other poses, like Cat and Cow (see next section), Child's Pose or Downward Facing Dog Pose. Although it seems simple, just being on hands and knees, there's a bit more subtlety to Table Pose. Let's practice it!

Come to your mat and down to hands and knees, with your knees hip-width apart and your hips right over the knees and your hands shoulder-width apart and just below the shoulders. Spread your fingers nice and wide so you feel a little stretch on the skin of your palms, point your thumbs toward one another with your

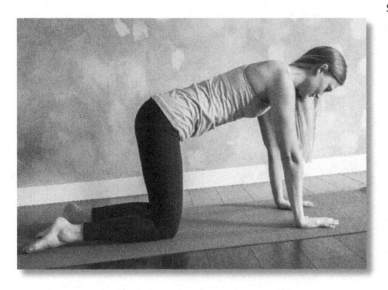

second finger pointing forward and press the mat away from you with both hands. Reach the crown of your head forward and keep your chin neutral so your neck is a natural extension of your spine. Press your tailbone back, flattening the spine and lift your navel slightly toward the spine, taking the little arch out of your low back. Enjoy three deep slow breaths, feeling the spine lengthen with each breath cycle. Continue breathing that way a few more times until you have a good sense of the shape of the body in the Pose: straight flat back, neck and head parallel to the mat, legs bent 90 degrees at the hips, knees bent so the shins are parallel to the mat and arms straight and reaching directly down to the mat. When you feel that you've got the shape, come out of the Pose.

Section 3 – Curved Body Poses

Remember that the curved body shape comes in three different variations: with the spine curved to the side (either right or left), spine rounded forward (usually with chin on sternum) and with the spine arched back (usually with the chin lifted up and away from the sternum). In this section we'll practice ten different poses that you'll often encounter in a yoga class and that represent each of the curved body shape variations.

Crescent Moon Pose *(Ashta Chandrasana)*

This Pose mimics the shape of a crescent moon, creating a long and wide arc from the feet on the mat to the arms stretching up to the sky. Notice that the arc

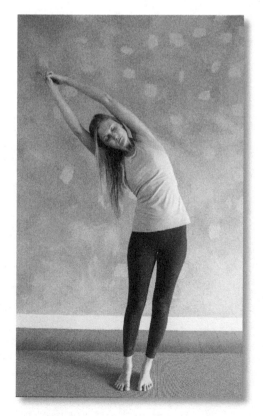

isn't limited to the torso, but continues into the arms and legs. Crescent Moon Pose lengthens one side of the body more than the other and results in a classic curved body shape.

Begin on your mat facing forward in Mountain Pose with your feet parallel to one another and about hip width, or even a little wider, apart. Inhale and reach both arms up and overhead, stretching the fingertips toward the sky with your arms parallel and your palms facing each other. Lengthen through the right side more than the left by pressing down on your right foot and reaching the right hand up a little more than the left. Taking care not to compress the left side body, allow your hips to slide to the right and at the same time reach your arms over to the left, allowing an arc to come into your entire body. You'll feel more of your weight coming into the left foot than the right which is fine. Check your alignment, making sure your feet, hips, shoulders, head and arms are all in the same plane, as though your movement was confined by two panes of glass about a foot apart and then pause for a few breaths, noticing that the spine is curved deeply to the left. Engage your core muscles even more deeply as you slowly bring your body back to center. Inhale and re-extend up toward the sky before exhaling as you move to the other side.

An option that will give you a little different feel in the Pose, as shown in the picture on the last page, is to interlace your fingers, press your palms together, point your index fingers and reach them up to the sky. This helps your body extend up and out of the shoulders and upper back.

Gate Pose *(Parighasana)*

Gate Pose is the second of our side curving poses. Because the knee of the lengthening side of the body is on the mat and the other leg is straight and providing support for the curve, Gate Pose will allow an even deeper side stretch than Crescent Moon Pose. Remember to keep your whole body in the same plane so that there's no twisting – just curving to the side.

Let's begin by kneeling on the mat with your hips directly above your knees, the shoulders over the hips and your head centered on your shoulders. Extend both arms up and overhead, reaching your fingertips to the sky. Transfer the

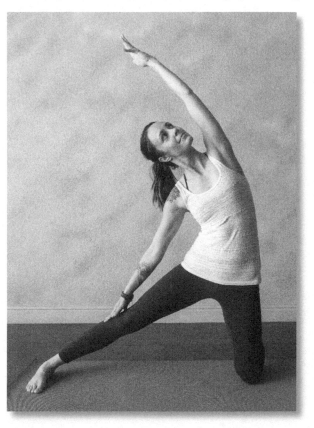

weight to your left knee as you lift the right knee off the mat and begin to straighten your right leg and reach it out to the side, setting the right foot down with your toes pointing the same direction your body is facing. Press into the pinkie toe of your right foot and roll your ankle to the outside. Reach your left arm up just a little bit higher than the right, lengthening all along the left side of your body and then drop your right hand down to the outside of your leg. Your hand will probably land just about at the knee. Now begin to reach your left arm up and over to the right, keeping as much length as you can in the right side body. Continue stretching your left hand up and along a wide arc to the right, feeling a deep stretch in your left side from the knee through the fingertips. You can allow your right hand to walk further down the outside of your right leg, keeping your arm straight. Once you've found your maximum side bend, take a few long deep breaths with your awareness on your left side body and notice the deep curve in your spine. When you're ready to come out of the Pose, engage the core more deeply (particularly the abs and the low back muscles) as you slowly rise up to the starting position. Bring your hands to your heart, pressing your palms lightly together, bend your right knee and bring that knee back to the mat about hip distance from your left knee. Let your hips drop to your heels and bring your palms to the top of the thighs. When you're ready, practice Gate Pose on the other side.

Standing Forward Fold Pose *(Uttanasana)*

Standing Forward Fold Pose features a rounded spine. Begin in Mountain Pose and then reach your arms up and overhead into Extended Mountain Pose, lengthening through the head, heart and fingertips. With the back flat begin to hinge at the hips and fold all the way over, bringing your hands down to the mat if

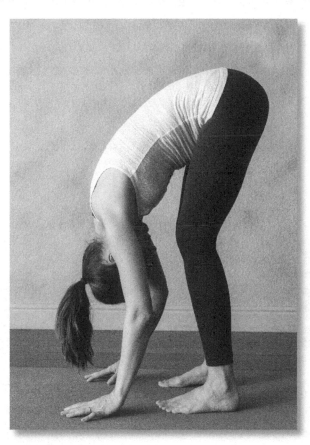

you can or at least stretching your fingertips toward your toes if you can't yet reach all the way down to the mat. You'll notice at some point as you're folding down that your low back will want to round. Go ahead and allow that to happen. If your hamstrings feel tight, bend your knees a bit. Be sure to release your neck muscles so you're not holding your head up. Allow the top of your head to reach down toward the mat. Finally, bring your weight into your toes (so you're not sitting back on your heels) by bringing your hips forward so they're right over your heels.

Take a few breaths and notice the rounding of the back, especially the low back. When you're ready to come out of the Pose, rise by rounding the back even more deeply as you keep your chin resting on your sternum and drag your hands up the outside of your legs and return to Mountain Pose.

Seated Forward Fold Pose *(Paschimottanasana)*

Seated Forward Fold Pose is the same shape as Standing Forward Fold Pose, except that it's done in a different spatial orientation. Begin seated on your mat with your legs straight and parallel to one another and all ten toes pointing straight up. Sit up tall, allowing the spine to lengthen, feeling both sitting bones pressing into the mat. Your chin is in a neutral position, neither lifting up away from the sternum nor pressing down toward the sternum. Inhale and reach your arms up and overhead, stretching your fingertips to the sky with the palms facing one another. Keep your back flat as you begin to hinge at the hips instead of bending

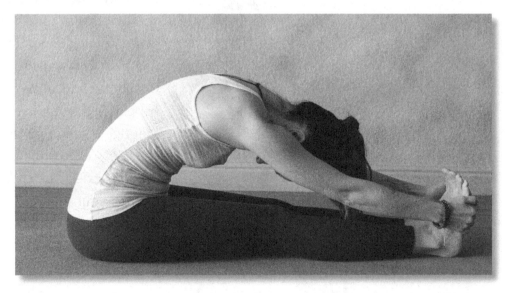

at the waist and reach your fingertips toward your toes. Hinge as far forward as you can with a flat back and then allow your back to round as your forehead comes down toward your knees or shins. If your hamstrings feel tight, you can bend your knees a little, which should release the hamstrings. Take the time to enjoy at least five breaths, lengthening through the crown of your head with each inhale and releasing down a little farther with each exhale. Notice that your spine is curved forward from the tailbone to the mid-back. When you're ready to come out of the Pose, bring your chin to the chest (if it's not already there) and round your back as you rise, coming back to Staff Pose.

Child's Pose – Knees Together Variation *(Balasana)*

Child's Pose with the knees together is the third of our poses featuring a rounded back. We practiced a version of Child's Pose with the straight body shaped poses. For this version, the back will round. Begin kneeling with the knees close together, the hips resting on the heels and your palms resting on your thighs. Start to slowly lower your torso forward toward the mat, eventually letting it rest on your thighs. Reach your arms back behind you and flip your palms so they face up and the back of the hands rest on the mat behind you. Relax your shoulders toward the

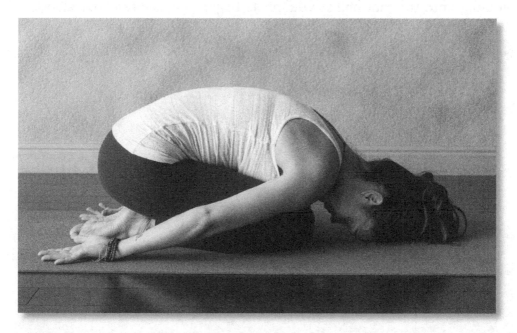

mat so they round over the outside of your knees. Let your forehead rest on the mat if it reaches (let it rest on a block if it doesn't reach down to the mat) and allow your chin to tuck, moving toward your sternum. Take a few breaths, noticing that your back is rounded from the tailbone to the base of your head. When you're ready to come out of the Pose, keep the back rounded as you rise to kneeling.

Cobra Pose *(Bhujangasana)*

Cobra Pose is another curved body shape and is the first of our curved body shaped poses where the spine bends backward. The Pose gets its name because it looks like a cobra reaching its head up to sense the world around it. Begin by lying face down on the mat. Untuck your toes so the toenails are resting on the mat and lengthen through both legs. Bring your hands right under your shoulders and hug your elbows in toward the body instead of flaring them out to the sides. Press your pubic bone into the mat and as you inhale begin to straighten your elbows a bit,

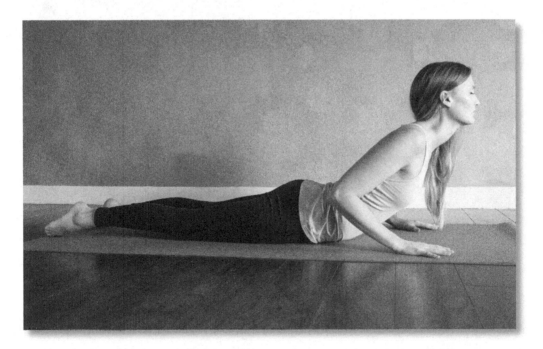

moving into a backbend and hugging your shoulder blades together and into your back. Reach your heart up, your ears away from your shoulders and allow the crown of your head to rise up toward the sky. Keep your neck long and try to avoid bunching up the skin on the back of your neck. Think about lengthening your front body, all the way from your big toes, through the front of the legs, the belly, the heart space and your head. Stay in the Pose for several breaths and when you're ready to come out of the Pose, exhale and lower down to the prone position with your belly on the mat.

   Variation. Sphinx Pose (Salamba Bhujangasana) is similar to Cobra Pose. The main difference is that in Sphinx Pose the elbows rest on the mat right below the shoulders and the forearms are kept parallel with the palms facing down. Begin Sphinx Pose in the same way as Cobra Pose, but instead of placing your hands below your shoulders, bring your elbows directly under the shoulders, place your

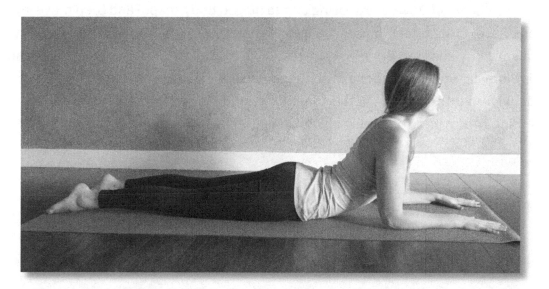

forearms parallel to one another with your palms on the mat. Lengthen the front of your body, just like Cobra Pose. The navel may lift a little off the mat, but the belly below the navel will rest on the mat. As you continue to lengthen up through the crown of your head (keeping the chin level), you'll feel a stretch come into the lower torso just above the navel. Press the heart forward and allow a deep backbend to emerge. When you're ready, come out of the Pose on an exhale.

Upward Facing Dog Pose *(Urdhva Mukha Svanasana)*

Upward Facing Dog is a very common pose you'll probably do in every yoga class, often as a transition between Plank Pose and Downward Facing Dog in a Vinyasa flow. While many yoga practitioners consider the Pose only as a transition, I love to remember it's a destination – a place to dwell for a while without hurrying into Downward Facing Dog.

Let's begin in Downward Facing Dog (a hinged body shape) and then move into Plank Pose, bringing the hips down into alignment with the shoulders and heels (a straight body shape). Bring your knees down to the mat and then the chest and chin, moving into a backbend in the manner of an inchworm, with your butt still reaching up into the air. At the same time, untuck your toes so the toenails are pressing lightly into the mat. Now glide your hips forward, press both hands into

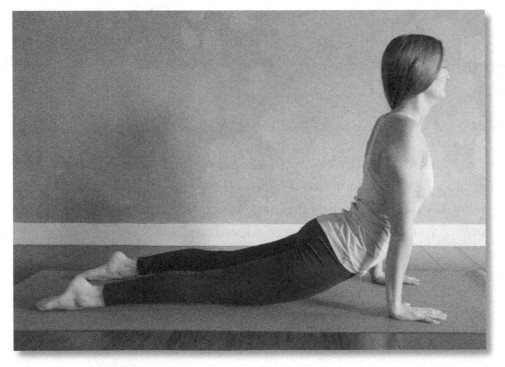

the mat, straighten the elbows and press the mat away from you with both hands. Reach your ears away from your shoulders, lifting your heart and lengthening through the front body, the neck and the crown of your head, and bring your shoulder blades together and hug them into your back. Finally, press through the toes, engaging the leg muscles and bringing your knees, shins and thighs off the mat. Your chin can either be level so your gaze is directly forward or, if you can do so without tension, lift your chin away from your chest and allow your gaze to rise up toward the sky. Enjoy a few breaths in the pose, feeling the deep arching of the spine as you continue to press your hands into the mat. When you're ready to come out of the Pose, first bring your chin down so it's level (if you lifted it up), then come back to Plank, tuck your toes, engage your core deeply and lift your hips into Downward Facing Dog Pose.

Locust Pose *(Salabhasana)*

Locust Pose is another backward curving shaped pose. It's done with the belly on the mat and the Pose is more about lengthening than it is about deep back bending, although the curved body shape, with the spine arching back, is unmistakable. There are a variety of different ways the arms are positioned in Locust Pose. We'll start with the most common arm position and then cover the different options in variations, below.

Begin lying down on the mat, as in Cobra Pose. Allow your arms to rest straight and long by your sides with your palms facing down. On an inhale, lift your head, shoulders, heart, hands, thighs, knees and your feet off the mat. Stretch your toes and fingertips toward the back of your mat and reach your forehead forward toward the front of your mat, lengthening through your entire body. Don't worry too much about lifting your head or feet up high. Concentrate instead on length.

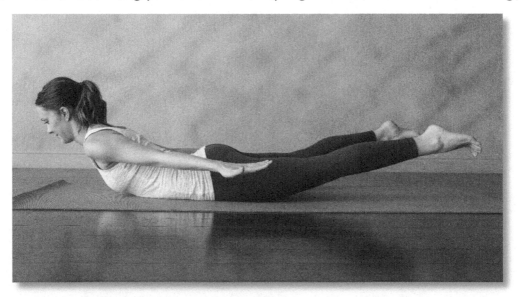

Try to keep your neck long, not bunching up the skin on the back of your neck. Stay in the Pose for a few breaths, noticing that when you inhale your body will rise up just a little and as you exhale it drops down a bit. Don't fight the rising and falling.

Just go with it. I call this riding the breath. When you're ready to come out of Locust Pose gently lower all the way down on an exhale.

Variations. There are several different arms positions that are commonly practiced in Locust Pose, each of which will give the Pose a little bit different feel.

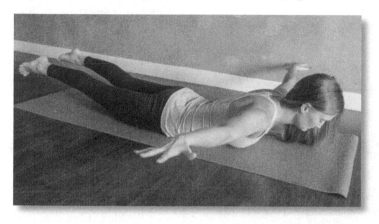

The first option is to bring your arms out to the side with the palms facing down, the Airplane Variation. As you inhale into the Pose, lift your hands off the mat and keep your hands level with your shoulders. Perhaps as you rise and fall with your breath in the Pose you can imagine yourself flying over a favorite landscape.

Another variation has the arms reaching forward from the shoulders, as if doing a full body stretch with the palms facing down (or with the palms facing one another as shown in the picture below). This variation will probably feel more

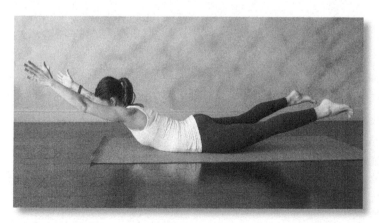

challenging to the core than any of the others. Begin as described above, but with your arms parallel and reaching forward, palms facing or down. As you rise into the Pose, lift your hands at the same time you lift your shoulders up. Stretch through your fingertips, reaching them forward and lengthening all the way along the body from the toes through the fingertips. Keep the gaze mostly down or just slightly forward and try to avoid lifting your chin too far away from your chest.

In the final variation, the arms begin in the same position as described above for the main Pose, long and by your sides. From there, lift your hands and bring

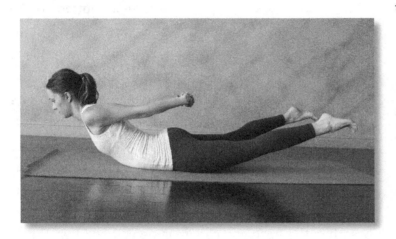

them together behind the back, interlacing your fingers, pressing your palms together and straightening your elbows. Rise into the Pose and lift your hands off your back, stretching your knuckles toward your heels. This will create a deeper backbend and bring the shoulder blades closer together than the other variations. Even with the deeper backward curving spine, keep your focus on lengthening the body from the toes stretching toward the back of your mat to the forehead and heart reaching forward.

Bridge Pose *(Setu Bandha Sarvangasana)*

Like Cobra Pose, Upward Facing Dog Pose and Locust Pose, Bridge Pose is a curved body pose with the spine curving backward into an arch. However, Bridge Pose is oriented face up. Bridge Pose is often encountered near the end of a yoga class, but is occasionally done at the beginning of class.

Begin by lying on your back on the mat with your arms long and by your sides, palms facing down. Bend your knees and bring the soles of your feet to the mat about hip-width apart with your heels under your knees. Ground into both feet equally with the weight distributed evenly between the heels and the balls of your feet. Inhale and press into both feet, lifting your hips as you press the back of your arms into the mat. Let your hips rise until you feel your spine beginning to curve backward into an arch. Lift the hips higher if you like, creating a deeper backward

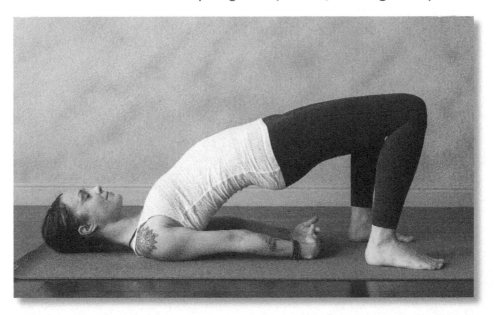

curve in the spine, lifting your heart up and creating length between the pubic bone and the sternum. You can bring your hands together behind your back, interlacing your fingers and pressing your forearms and the outside edges of the hands into the mat while straightening the elbows and stretching the knuckles toward your heels, bringing the shoulder blades closer together on the back and deepening the back bend. Take at least three breaths and when you're ready to come out of the Pose, exhale and release your hands if the fingers were interlaced and slowly lower your spine to the mat one vertebra at a time. When your tailbone lands on the mat, inhale and bring your knees to your chest, wrap your forearms or hands around your knees and give yourself a nice big hug, bringing your forehead to your knees if you like. Then exhale and release the back of your head and feet to the mat, coming back to the position you started in.

Crescent Lunge Pose *(Anjaneyasana)*

Crescent Lunge Pose is another of the curved body shaped poses. It is done with the body in an upright orientation and the spine curves backward into an arch. It is asymmetrical in the lower body because the left and right legs are in different positions, but symmetrical in the upper body. With the back knee resting on the mat, called a <u>Low</u> Crescent Lunge, the Pose deeply stretches the hip flexor muscles (the Psoas and the Iliacus).

Begin in Table Pose on hands and knees. Transfer the weight to the right knee and step the left foot forward so it ends up between the hands. Ground into the left foot, making sure your weight is distributed evenly between the ball and heel

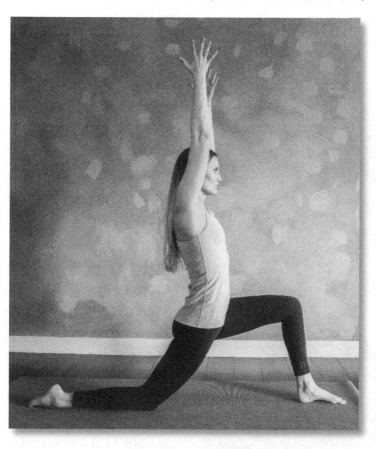

of the left foot. Pad the right knee if you need to by doubling the mat or using a blanket if you need to cushion that knee. Press into the left foot, lift your hands off the mat and reach your fingertips to the sky, straightening the arms. Press your hips forward, bending the left knee even more deeply (if the knee moves in front of the toes, come out of the Pose and step the left foot forward about six inches), and reach the heart, head and hands up to the sky.

Check in with the hips and make sure your hips are squared to the front of the mat. If you need to, square your hips by pressing your right hip forward and the left hip back. Now begin to notice the curved body shape emerging in the Pose, feeling the arch in your back. Soften your shoulders and reach your ears away from your shoulders. If it feels ok, you can lift your chin away from your sternum, deepening the backward curve, and reach your hands up and back. Keep lifting your heart toward the sky so your spine is curving consistently from your tailbone to your neck and you're not dumping into the low back. When you're ready to come out of Crescent Lunge, bring your shoulders back over your hips, take the backward curve out of your spine and bring your hands down to the mat on either side of your left foot. Flatten your back and step your left knee back to meet the right in Table Pose. When you're ready, perform the Pose on the other side.

Variation. High Crescent Lunge. Another way to do Crescent Lunge is with the back knee off the mat instead of resting on the mat. This variation usually feels

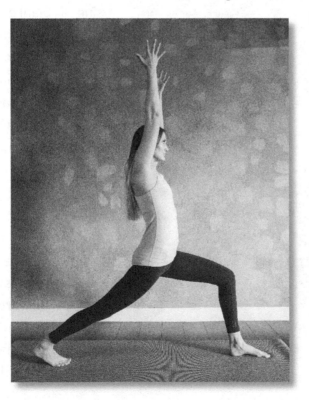

more energetic and engages the leg and core muscles in a little bit different way. Begin as you did for the Low Crescent Lunge by stepping your left foot forward between your hands from Table Pose and stepping the right foot back, tucking the toes and straightening your right leg. Instead of bringing the right knee to the mat, keep it lifted off the mat as you press back on the heel of the right foot. Grounding into the sole of the left foot, rise up and reach your arms overhead with your fingertips reaching for the sky. Press your hips forward with the left knee bent up to 90-degrees, feeling a deep stretch come into the hip muscles on the right side. If your left knee moves in front of the toes, come out of the Pose and step your left foot forward about six inches and then return to the Pose. If you feel unbalanced or wobbly in the Pose, move your left foot off to the left a few inches, widening your stance. Proceed as described above for the Low Crescent Lunge.

Warrior I Pose *(Virabhadrasana I)*

Warrior I, like Crescent Lunge, is an upright oriented curved body pose with the spine bending backward into an arch. Notice that it's also asymmetrical in the lower body and symmetrical in the upper body. You may be wondering whether Warrior I isn't the same pose as High Crescent Lunge. And for the most part, you'd be right. The only difference, which you'll see if you look closely at the pictures is that in Warrior I the heel of the back foot comes down to the mat and the toes on the back foot point off to the side about 35 degrees. In High Crescent Lunge, on the other hand (or foot), you're standing on the ball of the back foot and the toes are pointed forward. Although this may seem like a small change, it changes the

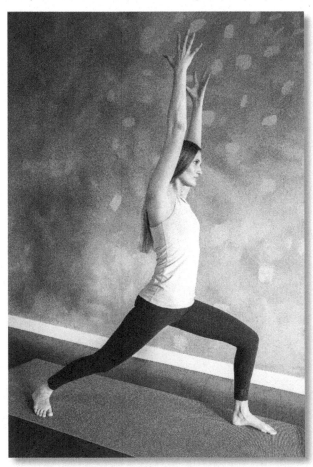

dynamics and feeling of the Pose quite a bit. Warrior I opens the groin muscles more than High Crescent Lunge and High Crescent Lunge emphasizes the hip flexor muscles more than Warrior I does.

We're going to come into Warrior I in a different way than we did for Crescent Lunge (and you can use this for the entry into Crescent Lunge too). Begin in Mountain Pose at the back of your mat. Step the left foot forward 3-4 feet and to the left about six inches, making sure the toes of your left foot point forward and grounding into the heel as well as the ball of the right foot. Bring the heel of your right foot to the mat so the toes of the right foot point about 35 degrees to the right, approximately toward the upper left corner of the mat. Bend your left knee (up to 90 degrees) and extend your arms up overhead, reaching your heart, head and fingertips toward the sky. Keep your right leg straight and strong and roll the ankle toward the back of the mat, pressing your pinkie toe into the mat. Now check in with your hips to make sure they're square to the front of the mat. You may want to bring your hands to your hips at this point and you'll probably need to nudge the right hip forward and pull the left hip back. When you're done squaring your hips, reach your hands back up overhead. As you press your hips forward a bit more, make sure you keep your shoulders over your hips and avoid leaning forward (or leaning back). Check in with your shoulders and make sure they're square to the front of the mat, just like the hips. Now take a few breaths and lift your heart a little bit higher as you begin to notice the backward curve in the spine, which may be a little more subtle than you experienced in Crescent Lunge Pose. If you're comfortable and stable in the Pose you can allow a deeper backbend, perhaps reaching your arms back so your biceps move behind your ears. You can even bring your hands together overhead if you like, interlacing your fingers. When you're ready to come out of the Pose, bring your hands down to the mat on either side of your left foot, transfer the weight to your hands and step your left foot back to meet the right in Plank Pose. Then release your knees to the mat. When you're ready, return to Mountain Pose and practice Warrior I on the other side by stepping the right foot forward.

Cow/Cat Flow

We finish this Chapter and our exploration of specific poses with something a little different. Cow Pose (Bitilasana) and Cat Pose (Marjaryasana) are almost always done together in a flow and rarely done separately. Both, of course, are curved body shapes. Cow Pose is a backbending pose, with the back arching and the spine curving backward, and Cat Pose is a deep back rounding pose, with the spine curving forward.

Begin the flow on hands and knees in Table Pose. Take a deep breath in as you drop your belly down, lift your chin away from your chest, press your heart forward

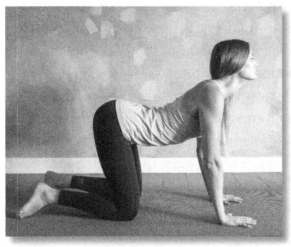

and imagine you're lifting your tailbone away from your knees. Keep the curved shape as you gently breathe in and out a few times, just noticing the deep arching back. Next, breathe in deeply and then exhale as you transition back through Table Pose, bringing your chin to your chest, pressing your hands into the mat, rounding your back, tucking your tailbone and pressing your forehead toward your thighs. Pause for a moment in Cat Pose, gently

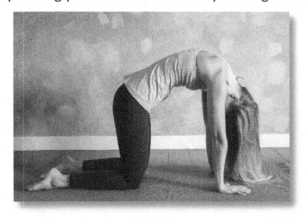

breathing in and out with your awareness on your spine and noticing the forward curve of the spine. As you breathe in, transition back to Cow Pose and then exhale into Cat Pose. Continue flowing through Cow and Cat a few more times, allowing your eyes to close and bringing your awareness to the bending and flexing of your spine, always inhaling to Cow Pose and exhaling to Cat Pose. Once you have the feeling of the flow, come back to a neutral spine in Table Pose, completing the flow.

Chapter 7 – Conclusion

The practice of yoga can be truly transformational and life-changing. Because of your diligence in working through the Practices in this book and all the specific poses we explored in Chapter 6, your mind and your body working together have a good understanding of the basics of the postural yoga practice. In a real way, yoga has already changed how you relate to and interact with your body. You know the basic shape your body will assume, straight, hinged at the hips or curved, in any yoga pose you've learned so far and the many more you will learn as you continue with your practice. You can also recognize that the three different body shapes can be oriented in space in different ways and that each orientation will result in a different yoga pose. Finally, you've learned that your arms, legs, torso and neck may be bent and twisted in different ways in a yoga pose and you definitely have the skills now to recognize how each part is positioned in each yoga pose. Equally important, you've gained deep new insight into how your body works and what it's capable of. You can tell the difference between holding your back straight or rounding or arching. As you learn new poses in the future, be sure to apply the skills you've learned in this book by asking yourself questions like:

- Is my body straight, hinged at the hips or curved in the pose?
- How is my body oriented in space in the pose?
- Are each of the knees and elbows bent or straight?
- How are the legs and arms positioned in the shoulder and hip joints?
- What in the pose is symmetrical and what's asymmetrical?
- Are the torso and neck twisted in the pose and if so, how?

What lies ahead for you are yoga classes where the teacher will guide you through specific poses, many of which you've already learned, linked together in a sequence.

There are many different places you can practice yoga and lots of styles of yoga for you to experience. You'll find scores of different types of classes, from gentle to vigorous, heated and not, emphasizing props or not, with devotional components like chanting or mostly stripped of devotional content, of different lengths, appealing to different experience levels and so on and so on. Try everything you can. Some may appeal to you and some may not. Sample a variety before you settle into any one style or type of practice. Tune into what your body is telling you and recognize that one type of class may appeal to you one day and another might feel better at a different time. For example, some days I really feel like an energetic and physically demanding practice and other days I want something more gentle and restorative.

If you belong to a gym, they probably have yoga classes you can take. There may be rec centers in your area that offer yoga classes as well. There are many studios dedicated solely to yoga or that offer yoga classes in addition to Pilates, tai chi, qi gong and the like. Most dedicated yoga studios offer a free or reduced-price trial period for you to see if the studio and its teachers are a "fit" for you. Take advantage of those opportunities to find a comfortable home, a place where you feel safe, supported and welcome.

You can find many classes online as well. While these have their place, I'd suggest that as a beginner you make the effort to attend in person classes as much as possible. A skilled teacher in a live class will be able to help you by pointing out misalignments you may not notice when you're first starting out. As you practice more and more, you'll begin to notice such things on your own. But when you're new to the practice having a teacher there to help you will be more than worth the effort and cost. There's also a completely different energy in an in-person class than in a video you do in your living room or basement on your own. You'll hear others breathing and feel their practice. It changes the experience of yoga to do it in a group. Finally, a skilled teacher will adjust the class based on what the teacher is observing in the students, maybe slowing it down or speeding it up or changing up the poses in the class based on the dynamic and changing needs of that particular group of students. You obviously aren't going to get that if you're just watching a video.

You can make of the practice of yoga whatever you like. If you practice solely to reap the benefits to your physical body arising from movement and breath, Yoga will reward you a hundred times over with a vigorous and youthful body, strong muscles, supple joints and improved balance. If you wade more deeply into the waters of Yoga you will find that movement can be meditative and will calm the mind and provide insights into what and who you are. Yoga is endless and without boundaries and you can explore it for the rest of your life.

In Chapter One I mentioned the Yoga Sutra by Patanjali, one of the foundational texts of Yoga. Although no one is sure when it was written, it's probably at least 2,000 years old. It consists of 196 verses, including these:

> *Sthira sukham āsanam (the postures of [yoga] should embody steadiness and ease)*
> *Prayatna śaithilya Ananta samāpatti bhyām (this occurs as all effort relaxes and coalescence arises, revealing that the body and the infinite universe are indivisible)*
> *Tato dvaṅdva an abhighātaḥ (then one is no longer disturbed by the play of opposites)[1]*

These three verses from the second of four sections of the Yoga Sutra are all Patanjali tells us about the postures – the asana. It is from this small seed that the robust practice of yoga asana has blossomed. Today there are millions of practitioners around the world and thousands joining the ranks every week. My aim in this book has been a simple one: to make Yoga more accessible to everyone, beginners and seasoned practitioners alike, by simplifying how the poses are thought of and understood. I hope you have found this book helpful in guiding you to the practice of Yoga and that you may embody Patanjali's ideal of practicing with both strength and ease and fostering harmony among body and mind.

---

[1] Translation by Chip Hartranft.

About the Author

Garry Appel lives and teaches Yoga full time in Denver, Colorado. Garry holds the E-RYT designation from the Yoga Alliance. *Learning Yoga* is Garry's first book on Yoga. You can connect with him on Facebook and visit his website at GarryAppel.com, where you can find other writings and share in Garry's other interests.

Made in the USA
Middletown, DE
11 June 2019